"The editors of this remarkable book have forged their ideas and concepts with an assembled group of inspired and engaging authors. Their contributions are rooted in clinical work and deep theoretical understanding. This book is not only a blueprint for clinicians and students alike but will stand as a reference in defining the discussion of the identity of psychoanalytic psychotherapy, present and future."

— **Hansjorg Messner M.A, EFPP board member, BPC and senior BPF member**

"A multi-voiced, well-articulated book, with diverse theoretical and clinical approaches but with the common denominator of the specific methodological training of Freudian psychoanalysis in its various forms and the passion for good work. In a dynamic balance between attention to the confusing inconveniences of the civilisation of our times and a firm basic trust in our basic paradigms, it offers a testimony and a point of reference for teaching activity and daily clinical practice as well as for a broader vision on the ethical role of a talking therapy in today's society."

— **Simona Argentieri, psychiatrist, psychoanalyst, Member of Associazione Italiana di Psicoanalisi**

"This book focuses on the development of psychoanalysis and psychoanalytic psychotherapy from a contemporary scientific and cultural perspective. The authors, rather than look once again at how to differentiate those above, move their attention to the new and stimulating contributions on the psychotherapeutic theory and technique. Change and Identity are the key words leading the reader through a fascinating journey inside the clinical practice."

— **Cristina Călărășanu, psychoanalytic psychotherapist, EFPP Vice President and Chair of the Couple and Family Section**

W0234900

Psychoanalytic Psychotherapy Between Identity and Change

Psychoanalytic Psychotherapy Between Identity and Change reconsiders psychoanalytic psychotherapy for contemporary contexts. This book stems from several years of study and research and aims to offer pragmatic and innovative working tools. The contributors approach psychoanalytic psychotherapy as its own practice with distinctive features and benefits to patients. Each chapter considers the history of the field as well as today's social and cultural context, presenting innovative approaches based on each author's clinical experience. A range of settings and applications, including online therapy, artistic expression, and psychotherapy with personality disorders, are explored.

This book will be of interest to psychoanalytic psychotherapists and psychoanalysts in practice and in training.

Luigia Cresti is a psychologist, and adult and child psychotherapist. She is a Founder Member and former President of the Florentine Association of Psychoanalytic Psychotherapy (AFPP) and a former European Delegate for EFPP. She is also Editor-in-Chief of the scientific journal, *Contrappunto.*

Isabella Lapi is a psychologist, child and adult psychotherapist, and President of AFPP. She is the former Chief Consultant of the Mental Health Department, an expert in training of medical staff, and a specialist in bioethics, perinatality and mourning.

The EFPP Monograph Series

Series Editor: Anne-Marie Schlösser

A series of Monographs produced in conjunction with the European Federation for Psychoanalytic Psychotherapy (EFPP). Each volume brings together writings on a particular topic by authors from several European countries. The EFPP promotes communication and discussion between psychotherapists across national boundaries in the child and adolescent, adult, family and group sections of the organisation, through its conferences and seminars on topics of interest in contemporary psychoanalytic psychotherapy. The organisation represents some 13,000 psychoanalytic psychotherapists in twenty-two countries in Western, Central and Eastern Europe and is concerned with many matters which are relevant to the profession, such as training and registration.

Recent titles in the series include:

Psychoanalytic Psychotherapy of the Severely Disturbed Adolescent
Edited by Dimitris Anastasopoulos, Margot Waddell and Effie Lignos

Families in Transformation
A Psychoanalytic Approach
Edited by Anna Maria Nicolo, Pierre Benghozi and Daniela Lucarelli

A Psychoanalytic Exploration of Social Trauma
The Inner Worlds of Outer Realities
Edited by Cristina Călărăşanu, Ulrich Schultz-Venrath and Hansjorg Messner

Psychoanalytic Psychotherapy Between Identity and Change
Edited by Luigia Cresti and Isabella Lapi

For further information about this series please visit:
https://www.routledge.com/The-EFPP-Monograph-Series/book-series/
KARNACEFPPPM

Psychoanalytic Psychotherapy Between Identity and Change

Edited by
Luigia Cresti and Isabella Lapi

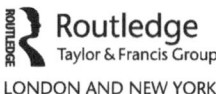
Routledge
Taylor & Francis Group

LONDON AND NEW YORK

Designed cover image: © "Change" by Giovanni Pibiri

First published 2025
by Routledge
4 Park Square, Milton Park, Abingdon, Oxon OX14 4RN

and by Routledge
605 Third Avenue, New York, NY 10158

Routledge is an imprint of the Taylor & Francis Group, an informa business

Published in Italian in 2022 as La psicoterapia psicoanalitica tra identità e cambiamento.

British Library Cataloguing-in-Publication Data
A catalogue record for this book is available from the British Library

ISBN: 978-1-032-67371-4 (hbk)
ISBN: 978-1-032-67368-4 (pbk)
ISBN: 978-1-032-67372-1 (ebk)

DOI: 10.4324/9781032673721

Typeset in Times New Roman
by Taylor & Francis Books

Note on translation

The English translation has been revised by Aldo Grassi and Luigia Cresti

Contents

Illustrations

Figures

Box

About the editors and contributors

Editors

Luigia Cresti is a psychologist and psychotherapist of children, adolescents and adults, is a founding member of AFPP, and a lecturer with training functions. She is the past President of AFPP and a former EFPP European Delegate. She is a specialist in Infant Observation methodology and its applications, with international recognition. She has conducted numerous training courses for socio-medical-educational practitioners and has published extensively in books and journals, presented numerous papers at universities, in national and international congresses and is Editor-in-Chief of the journal, *Contrappunto*.

Isabella Lapi is a psychologist and psychotherapist for minors and adults, an ordinary member of AFPP and trainer, and is the current AFPP President. She is also a specialist in Bioethics at the University of Florence and former Head of the mental health services of the USL Toscana Centro, Italy. She is dedicated to the training of practitioners in public and private institutions, and universities. Her research fields are care relationships, perinatality and mourning. She has published extensively in books and journals and is the Editor of *Contrappunto*.

Contributors

Cristina D. Canzio is an Italian-Argentinian clinical and social psychologist, and an ordinary member and lecturer with training functions of the AFPP. She is a psychotherapist specializing in systemic psychotherapy at the Mental Research Institute, Palo Alto, USA, and the Center of the Berkshires, Massachusetts, USA, specializing in Operational Group Analysis, with Armando J. Bauleo (IIPSA). She is a founding member of the Korinthos Institute of Florence for the Analysis of Affective Culture in Institutions. She directs the Hispano-American Section of the International Association of Art & Psychology. A founding member and President of the Italian Association of Multifamily Groups (AIGM), she is also a painter.

Corrado D'Agostini is a psychiatrist, geriatrician and psychotherapist and the former Professor of Clinical Psychology in the Faculty of Medicine at the University of Florence, Italy. He is an ordinary member and lecturer with training functions of the AFPP. The former head of the Villa dei Pini Nursing Home in Florence, he has gained extensive experience in the field of eating disorders and personality disorders. He has collaborated on an ongoing basis with the Nutrition Agency of the University of Florence, of which he was a co-founder. He is the author, editor and co-author of more than 80 publications and books on topics pertaining to psychodynamics.

Esmeralda Di Mauro is a child and adult psychologist and psychotherapist, an ordinary member and AFPP lecturer. She has worked for many years in residential communities for seriously ill, disabled and juvenile patients. She currently carries out her clinical work with adults and children both privately and at the Meyer Children's Hospital in Florence. A specialist in Infant Observation, her main area of interest is perinatal care.

Alfredina Fiori is a psychologist and psychotherapist, an ordinary member of the AFPP. She has worked for a long time in the public service of the USL Toscana Centro, Italy, dealing with adoption and family foster care paths, as well as juvenile protection, applying integrated actions of intervention in complex situations of distress. In this field she has promoted, in addition to the individual clinic, multidisciplinary work activities with self-help groups and outpatient clinics dedicated to adoptive parenting. A specialist in the psychotherapy of adolescents, she has been in charge of psychological listening and reception activities at the USL youth-oriented counselling centres.

Giulia Mercuriali is a psychologist and psychotherapist, an ordinary member of the AFPP, and a lecturer at the Child Psychotherapeutic Clinic, Italy. She is the founding member and treasurer of the Italian Association of Multifamily Groups (AIGM). One of her areas of interest is perinatal care. She works in Florence as a freelancer with children, adolescents, adults and multifamily groups.

Stefania Pampaloni is a psychologist and psychotherapist, and an ordinary member and lecturer at the AFPP post-graduate school. She conducts private psychotherapy and consults for public agencies on training, employment guidance and counselling, in research projects and surveys. She promotes the activities of the ASPIG Association, of which she is president, for the development of psychological sciences in the social and health fields, through psychological planning and counselling activities.

Cristina Pratesi is a psychologist and psychotherapist, an ordinary member of the AFPP, a lecturer with training functions, the scientific secretary, and former Director of the AFPP School of Specialization in Psychoanalytic Psychotherapy. She is a founding member of the Italian Association of Multifamily Groups (AIGM). She is the former head of a child and adolescent mental health service of the USL Toscana Centro, Italy. She is the author of scientific contributions in national and international publications. Her areas of interest are pregnancy, adolescence, bereavement and education.

Rosa Romano Toscani is a founding member of the Italian Society of Psychoanalytic Psychotherapy (SIPP), where she holds the role of teacher with training functions, a member of the EFPP (European Federation for Psychoanalytic Psychotherapy) and an ordinary member of the Italian Society of Psychoanalysis and Sándor Ferenczi Psychotherapy. She is also a member of the National Association for the Advancement of Psychoanalysis. She has written numerous scientific works and novels , some translated into French, *The Girl from Charlie's Café*.

Antonio Suman is a psychiatrist-psychotherapist, a founding member and former president of AFPP, and a lecturer with training functions. He is the past president of SIEFPP, the former coordinator of the Tuscany Section and currently a member of the SIMP Board, and is vice-president of the Florence Psychosomatic Training Institute (IFP). He participated in the Psychosomatic Unit of the Florence University Dermatology Clinic, and was a conductor of Balint Groups for general practitioners and hospital physicians. He has published numerous papers in Italian and foreign journals on psychoanalytic and psychosomatic psychotherapy topics.

Manuela Trinci is a psychologist, a child psychotherapist with psychoanalytic training, essayist, scholar of children's literature, and lives and works in Pistoia, Italy. She is a founding member and teacher of the "Dina Vallino" Scientific-cultural Association, and scientific contact in the scientific direction of the library of the Meyer Pediatric Hospital in Florence. She has had numerous publications in scientific journals and collaborations with newspapers, weeklies and magazines.

Foreword

Rosa Romano Toscani

Sigmund Freud, in "Ways of Psychoanalytic Therapy", stated:

> We are ready to admit the imperfections of our knowledge, to learn new
> things and to change our way of proceeding where it can be developed ...
> to re-examine the situation of our therapy ... to consider the new direc-
> tions in which it might develop ... The large-scale application of our
> therapy will oblige us to bind to a large extent the pure gold of analysis
> with the bronze of suggestion ... But whatever strength this psychother-
> apy will assume for the people, whatever elements will constitute it, it is
> certain that its most effective and significant skills will remain those bor-
> rowed from rigorous psychoanalysis and alien to all taken sides.
>
> (1918 [2001])

Reading today, more than a century later, Freud's words: "admitting imper-
fections", "learning new things", "mutating", "re-examining", "considering",
already immerses us "in medias res" in the book we are presenting.

Freud had foreseen that the future of psychoanalysis would lie not only in
the important theoretical assumptions, which are the foundations of the psychoanalytic discipline, but also in the comparison with the clinical aspects, in
the conscious and unconscious relationship that the therapist would create
with "that" patient, with the knowledge he would seek to have of his internal
world, of his defences, of his suffering and with the "whys" he would ask
himself. He had understood that the "most effective components ... borrowed
from psychoanalysis" would find other applications by extending the doc-
trine's efficacy into other equally rigorous fields.

By means of a dialectical crusade, Freud had sought to experience the
many states of being of the patient and the therapist, through the limited time
of the session, but also over the long course of the treatment, in which the
"reflecting" of the analytical couple would allow one to know and recognise
what is not known and not recognised.

A specific feature of psychoanalysis, and thus of psychoanalytic psychotherapy, if we refer to Freud's teachings, is the epistemological tension

which leads to asking questions, not taking for granted positions that one believes to have been achieved.

This book, *Psychoanalytic Psychotherapy Between Identity and Change*, edited by Luigia Cresti and Isabella Lapi, is situated in a furrow that has been traced for some time. As Luigia Cresti and Antonio Suman state in Chapter 1, the debate has been going on "since the early 1980s".

Indeed, Emanuel Berman (2019), in his beautiful book, *Il training impossibile* [*The Impossible Training*], reminds us that from a theoretical point of view, innovative aspects cannot originate from isolated minds, but can evolve in a "transitional space" (Winnicott, 1955) within a relationship, to develop a psychoanalysis ready for new challenges.

Clara Mucci (2019; 2020), moreover, considers "the human, ethical, philosophical assumptions … the warp and woof of the psychoanalytic fabric", the "glue, in my view, that can give lifeblood to a psychoanalysis in step with the times".

I am thinking of a wide-ranging training, already suggested by Freud when he argued that: "analytical teaching should include … extraneous subjects … history of civilisation, mythology, psychology of religions, literature" (1925 [2001]).

The acquisition of a psychoanalytic mind, and indeed, of "a psychoanalytic heart", cannot be satisfied with predictable questions and answers; it is not only important to ask what you "know" with respect to a given theory, but above all, who you "are".

This, in brief, is the message the authors wish to convey and it is what the Associazione Fiorentina di Psicoterapia Psicoanalitica (AFPP), which belongs to the European Federation for Psychoanalytic Psychotherapy (EFPP), has not only proposed, but has pursued with honesty of purpose in its statute since its foundation in 1979:

> to foster an in-depth ability to conduct the therapeutic relationship by following an organic programme that [takes] into account clinical activity, specific theoretical acquisitions and emotional experiences related to psychotherapeutic work and group activities … The theory to be referred to is the psychoanalytic one.

In the long interview, *Pensieri di uno psicoanalista irriverente. Guida per analisti e pazienti curiosi* [*A Guide for Analysts and Curious Patients*], Antonino Ferro's answer to the question about the difference between psychoanalysis and psychotherapy is:

> One could cite if not thousands, hundreds of theories in this regard. I would say that some difference exists, but I could not yet indicate what, and I like to add "yet" because there is the idea that one day we will know more … We do not know what the healing factors are … the real

healing is to make unconscious what is too much conscious, that is, to transform a too concrete reality into a reality that is possible to dream.

(2017)

It is from these kinds of reflections that the authors of this book have started, greatly extending the research on the subject. They raise many questions, seeking answers to the therapist's identity, his or her ability to meet challenges, the search for new technical tools and loyalty to psychoanalysis.

Indeed, Luigia Cresti and Isabella Lapi put in their introduction to a "Table of Thoughts" – as they have called their long-standing way of coming together to create a common thought – that type of thinking of which Berman (2019) speaks, which is generative of ideas and projects, and issues of vital importance for psychoanalysis and psychoanalytic psychotherapy.

I agree so much with this approach that I started my book, *Percorsi in psicoterapia psicoanalitica* [*Pathways in Psychoanalytic Psychotherapy*] (Romano Toscani, 2019) with the chapter entitled "Pensare insieme" [Thinking together]. And that is exactly what I also find in this chapter. When reading what Cresti and Suman have written in this book, one is struck by the personal and group pathways taken, the teachings received from eminent scholars such as D. Meltzer, A. Alvarez, F. Palacio-Espasa, A. Pazzagli, L. Di Cagno, or M. Ponsi, to name but a few, over time.

In addition to the cultural growth of the authors' associations, we feel it is necessary to highlight how much this book focuses on the path of psychoanalysis and psychoanalytic psychotherapy in the contemporary scientific and cultural landscape. Rather than discussing the age-old question of the differences between psychoanalysis and psychoanalytic psychotherapy, what interests us are the new and more stimulating contributions to psychotherapeutic theory and technique.

Defining psychoanalysis and distinguishing it from psychoanalytic psychotherapy already presented difficulties in 1953 at the Congress of the American Psychoanalytic Association, where an agreement on an acceptable definition seemed to be found (Rangell, 1954). Psychoanalysis was understood to be therapy in which the analysis of transference was central, whereas, in psychotherapy, transference is used rather than interpreted. For example, it should be noted that since psychotherapists chose to analyse transference and adopt analytical techniques in therapy at a frequency of one or two sessions per week (also thanks to the supervision of psychoanalysts called upon to carry out this task), the distinction between psychotherapy and psychoanalysis has further blurred (Rocchi and Di Volo, 2013).

In his speech at the international conference "Dalla mente di Edipo al volto di Narciso?" [From the Mind of Oedipus to the Face of Narcissus?], André Green stated:

However, I think Otto Kernberg is right: one must distinguish the theoretical level from the clinical level. Otto perfectly understood that the model of psychoanalytic treatment is an ideal model, it is the ideal to which the psychoanalyst tends. And if he later practises psychotherapy in all its various forms, he will always retain this ideal model of psychoanalysis as it was conceived by Freud.

(1983)

This book was born as a result of such debates, and from its very beginning we sense the direction in which the authors want to lead us, stating that psychoanalysis and psychoanalytic psychotherapy represent the North Star for each other:

[that] there is not a problem of hierarchies but of differences: [while] psychotherapy starts from the real towards the mental by including it more and more … psychoanalysis starts from the unmentalised limit by making it mental and tending towards the real.

(Pazzagli, 1992)

Psychoanalytic psychotherapy, while holding firmly to the assumptions of psychoanalysis, is articulated by giving fundamental importance to the transference-countertransference relationship, to the flexibility of the setting in relation to the patient (Gino and Romano Toscani, 1998), to the preliminary assessment of symptoms, to the variation of the transference in relation to the type of setting, to the aims of the treatment, to the attention to the real, to the body, to the different levels of symbolisation, to dreams, to the non-interpretive therapeutic factors, to the function of interpretation, to the space and time experienced in today's society and to the new technologies. It is impossible to ignore how social changes inevitably reflect on individuals and their way of living and "being in the world", on their pathologies, on their identities which, today, are increasingly declined in narcissistic spectrum pathologies, in a sense of indefinite malaise (Bollas, 2018).

In their dual role as "observers" and "actors" (Bion, 2013), given the fast and disruptive social changes, therapists find it more difficult to be in the therapeutic relationship, to create that transformative "we" (Lingiardi, 2019), and, therefore, areccalled to find new relational and interpretative tools. We are in a particular moment in the development of psychoanalysis, as psychoanalytic psychotherapy, its direct heir, has allowed that "field" work, that direct experience which is capable of changing and enriching traditional theoretical assumptions, offering "this secret art" more scope.

The intention, therefore, of the book *Psychoanalytic Psychotherapy Between Identity and Change* is to suggest topics for discussion, in-depth study and comparison with colleagues from other associations and training schools, even those that are geographically distant.

We know how warm and fruitful the relationship of the AFPP with the SIPP, the Italian Psychoanalytic Psychotherapy Society, has been since their respective constitutions because the two societies have the same training goals.

The authors, in their clinical practice, address the nature and principles of psychic change in patients, with more attention to therapeutic goals, the environmental context, non-verbal communication, more measured interpretations, and a different flexibility in accepting and treating "acting".

It also seems important to accept the statement that in psychotherapeutic treatment there can be "moments in which in psychoanalysis one works in the psychotherapeutic sense and in psychotherapy in the psychoanalytic sense". While the "psychoanalytic sense" may seem clearer, the psychotherapeutic one is still a work in progress, but this is its richness and, as S. Bolognini, quoted by Cresti and Suman, states: "Long gone are the days when psychoanalytic psychotherapy seemed to be a by-product of psychoanalysis and ... the former showed the great merit of recognizing the necessary adaptation to changing needs" (2019).

The theoretical contribution given to the term *containment* seems to me to be important, in all the authors who have worked to define it, starting with Klein (1950) up to the present day, distinguishing between therapeutic containment, internal and external, and, above all, specifically Luigia Cresti moves in this area with Chapter 2, "Non-interpretive therapeutic factors: containing functions in the therapeutic relationship".

Through the presentation of clinical situations, she revisits the concepts of rêverie, containment, and holding as a function of the therapeutic relationship by giving value to non-interpretive tools, such as the patient's need to be seen, deepening the notion of visual *enveloppe* on the part of the therapist, through the internal and external gaze, in a circular process of mutual and multiple mirroring.

Cresti pays much attention to the transformative function of the gazes meeting in psychoanalytic psychotherapy, in the mirroring of affects, in making the patient learn "the existence of emotions", in the voice "that envelops ... that warms ... that cradles" like a lullaby, to patients deprived of necessary maternal functions. Emphasising the musicality of the voice seems very important to me. I believe that identity and change are to be sought precisely in these "non-interpretive factors" and can also be found in the greater sensitivity and therapeutic capacity acquired through study and continuous confrontation with the theoretical foundations being "inside" and "holding or supporting". Unseen patients can find "gazes" that meet, "voices" that envelop and warm. A theme taken up by Isabella Lapi, in Chapter 2, entitled "The musicality of voice in online psychotherapic consultations", an important contribution made during the time of the pandemic: "a voice that filled the silence of solitude, that became object and subject, taking on the meaning of person when the perceptive aspect of the body was missing".

Freud in *The Ego and the Id* (1922 [2001]) had stated: "The Ego is first and foremost a bodily entity", highlighting the close link between psyche and body, but this important statement was later disregarded. Only recently has psychoanalysis, but above all psychoanalytic psychotherapy, been questioning and deepening the function of the body, not only as an entity belonging to the subject, but also in relation to its symbolic function and the role it plays in the therapeutic relationship. The focus on this topic, therefore, could not be missing in a chapter that poses innovative questions. Luigia Cresti takes charge in Chapter 3 of studying "The body in the therapeutic relationship", both by offering a theoretical excursus and by presenting clinical vignettes in which the body is "embodied" (Lemma, 2019).

The other clinical contributions, by other colleagues, show a body that is not accepted by the patient, a source of discomfort and suffering, a disabled body, which requires emotional contact, but also puts distance, and the therapist's body when she becomes pregnant, activating fantasies, the object of identifications and projections.

Chapter 4 by Isabella Lapi, "Gestures that touch, actions that heal", continues this exploration of other communication channels and thus other interpretative tools: perhaps we can no longer speak of interpretation, but of interpretations, using the plural, and it is more appropriate, in my view, to also speak of "listening".

The realm of psychoanalytic psychotherapy lies in that "in-between", in that exchange of deep experience, in the equivalence that is given and received, in the moment that separates content and word. The "listening", conscious and unconscious, precedes the interpretations that are not necessarily verbal expressions, and induces the therapist, as the authors of this book propose, to ask questions that do not suggest an end, so that human thought does not become locked in rigid schemes.

Also, in this work we see how the communication between therapist and patient opens up to other registers, such as touch, which can become a therapeutic tool or disturb the relationship, the embrace that conveys emotions of gratitude, as the author of the chapter points out.

It is necessary to find different words to construct, as I said before, the "we", words that caress, that "untie knots" and open up new ways of taking care. This, I believe, is the specifics of psychoanalytic psychotherapy; it is what the patient is asking for and it is the real answer that the therapist can and must give, in order to – to borrow Lapi's words – "sail to distant lands" and conquer a new and more appropriate emotional and mental set-up. The unconscious belongs to the internal world that is not realised, but manifests itself nonetheless.

We now move to another area, in defining patients with a non-integrated sense of identity through "Adaptations of technique in the psychotherapy of borderline patients". In Chapter 7, Corrado D'Agostini revisits the concept of the term *borderline*, on its way from being considered by Kernberg (1985) a personality organisation, by Grinker (1968) a syndrome, probably determined by social and cultural changes, by Spitzer and Endicott (1979) a personality disorder, to being defined by the PDM (*Psychodynamic Diagnostic Manual*) according to "four components consisting of the sense of identity … the quality of object relations, the level of defences and the reality examination". From considering the symptom as the central axis, the definition shifted to the function of the internal components of thought and the ability to exercise them. This conception widened the understanding of this pathology, considering it a deficit of mentalisation, a difficulty in accessing the symbol, the existence of split thinking areas produced by deficiencies in early childhood care with neurobiological impairments (Shore, 2012).

The theoretical vision has enriched the clinician with wide-ranging tools, but what emerges from D'Agostini's exposition of the clinical case is the quality of the relationship offered to the patient, the containment, the emotional intensity of acceptance, the ability to listen, the "calming and ordering rhythm" of the sessions, but also the "authoritative firmness" necessary with certain psychic situations in which the limits are lax or non-existent.

What we feel is important to highlight in this book is the human and professional quality of the authors who combine theoretical expertise and relational qualities. Thus, when "patients [are] unable to dream", it becomes "necessary to have a shared language and code of reading, helping the patient to transform suffering into a narrative". In Chapter 6, Alfredina Fiori and Cristina Pratesi show a particular sensitivity with narcissistic patients who are not always able to "tolerate intrusion [as] not everything can be said directly". The cases presented show the therapist's ability not only in providing classic interpretations, but also in approaching the patients by widening the field with "inspired interpretations" of their history, their artistic and literary interests, even if they are modest.

The road to dreams opens up, creativity becomes a mediation between dreaming and waking and the "dream [appears] a project, an itinerary, a movement … the therapist is the bridge that allows the passage between bodily reality and psyche, between sleep and wakefulness".

In Chapter 5, Stefania Pampaloni ventures into new territories for the patient, dealing with the therapist's dreams. The therapist is considered a subject who participates with her own mental representations in the patient's "unprocessed areas". A complex work that foregrounds the authenticity of the therapist, through language expansions that include her conscious and unconscious countertransference that she uses to understand the patient.

The therapist's dreams in supervision, according to Cristina Pratesi in Chapter 5, are along the same lines, albeit in different areas, and take the form of a further vision to stimulate thinking in a flexible and open manner in the trainee. In Chapter 8, the relationship between psychotherapy and artistic expression also makes Cristina Canzio think of "psychoanalytic psychotherapy as an opportunity … without aiming to create a beginning or an end, without concern for being … the therapist allows them to encounter that intermediate zone".

This seems to me ultimately the function of psychoanalytic psychotherapy. Green affirms:

> Different branches of knowledge could offer the psychoanalyst a field of investigation. The method that made it possible to highlight the manifestations of the unconscious would provide, if necessary, the means to demonstrate the fruitfulness of psychoanalysis' conceptions in fields that are far removed from the cure.
>
> (1983)

Only such a mental and emotional disposition allows one to go towards the West. In Chapter 9, Cristina Pratesi leads us to very stimulating reflections on the experience of *psychotherapy at a distance* which is not so much at a distance, since the psychotherapist's expertise, acquired over long years of training, nonetheless allows a meaningful and transformative relationship to be established.

"Teleanalysis" represents a revolutionary way of doing therapy, involving changes in the therapist and the patient. As Paul-Claude Racamier (1995) states, the psychoanalytic psychotherapist must continue to "search", to "dig", to explore new concepts and find new technical strategies. We invite at this point, in the reading of this book, to leave the reader the nourishment to be received.

Chapter 10, "… and the door closes". Just as a therapist, when the therapeutic encounter ends, puts himself in the mental condition of reconsidering the session, Antonio Suman traces a path of reflection, which has to do with keeping the patient in mind, even during his absence, in the conscious and unconscious presence that allows him to "dream of him". Suman suggests "One can rethink the session without writing: after all, even psychotherapy … is no less than psychoanalysis, 'a process based on thinking and rethinking, dreaming and redreaming, discovering and rediscovering'" (Ogden, 2009).

Albeit it is certain that we have presented our colleagues with a high scientific profile, we are, however, convinced, that such questions always await further answers.

References

Berman, E. (2019). *Impossible Training*. London: Routledge.

Bion, W. (2013). *Seminari italiani*. Milan: Raffaello Cortina.

Bollas, C. (2018). *Meaning and Melancholia: The Age of Bewilderment*. London: Routledge.

Bolognini, S. (2019). *Flussi vitali tra il Sé e il non Sè*. Milan: Raffaello Cortina.

Ferro, A. (2017). *Pensieri di uno psicoanalista irriverente*. Milan: Raffaello Cortina.

Freud, S. (1918 [2001]). Ways of Psychoanalytic Therapy. In J. Strachey (ed.), *The Standard Edition of the Complete Psychological Works of Sigmund Freud*, vol. XVII *(1917/1919)*. London: Hogarth Press.

Freud, S. (1922 [2001]). The Ego and the Id. In J. Strachey (ed.), *The Standard Edition of the Complete Psychological Works of Sigmund Freud*, vol. XX *(1920/1922)*. London: Hogarth Press.

Freud, S. (1925 [2001]). An Autobiographical Study. In J. Strachey (ed.), *The Standard Edition of the Complete Psychological Works of Sigmund Freud*, vol. XX *(1925/ 1926)*. London: Hogarth Press.

Gino, M. and Romano Toscani, R. (1998). *Ritmo e setting*. Rome: Borla.

Green A. (1983). *Narcissisme de vie, narcissisme de mort*. Paris: Les Éditions de Minuit.

Green, A. (2009). Un dialogo sulla differenza tra psicoanalisi e psicoterapia psicoanalitica International Conference "Dalla mente di Edipo al volto di Narciso?", *Psychotherapy and the Human Sciences*, XLIII(2): 215–234.

Grinker, R. (1968). *The Borderline Syndrome: A Behavioural Study of Ego-Function*. London: Basic Books.

Kernberg, O. (1985). *Borderline Condition and Pathological Narcissism*. New York: Jason Aronson.

Klein, M. (1950). *The Psychoanalysis of Children*. London: Hogarth Press.

Lemma, A. (2019). The Aesthetic Bond: The Patient's Use of the Analyst's Body and the Body of the Analysis Room. *Review of Psychoanalysis*, LXV(1): 107–127.

Lingiardi, V. (2019). *Io, tu, noi*. Turin: Utet.

Mucci, C. (2019). Prefazione. In R. Romano Toscani, *Percorsi in psicoterapia psicoanalitica*. Milan: FrancoAngeli.

Mucci, C. (2020). *Corpi borderline*. Milan: Raffaello Cortina.

Ogden, T.H. (2009). *Rediscovering Psychoanalysis: Thinking and Dreaming, Learning to Forget*. London: Routledge.

Pazzagli, A. (1992). Psicoterapia psicoanalitica. *Contrappunto*, 10: 9–19.

Racamier, P.C. (1995). *L'inceste et l'incestuel*. Paris: Dunod.

Rangell, L. (1954). Similarities and Differences Between Psychoanalysis and Dynamic Psychotherapy. *Journal of the American Psychoanalytic Association*, 2: 734–744.

Rocchi, C. and Di Volo, F. (2013). Psicoanalisi e psicoterapia psicoanalitica. Available at: www.spiweb.it (accessed 14 April 2022).

Romano Toscani, R. (2019). *Percorsi in psicoterapia psicoanalitica*. Milan: FrancoAngeli.

Shore, A.N. (2012). *The Science of the Art of Psychotherapy*. London: Norton & Co.

Spitzer, R. and Endicott, J. (1979). Justification for Separating Schizotypal and Borderline Personality Disorders. *Schizophrenia Bulletin*, 5(1): 95–104.

Winnicott, D.W. (1955). *Through Paediatrics to Psychoanalysis*. London: Tavistock Publications.

Preface

Manuela Trinci

"You see, doctor, I don't have anything to talk about," the melancholic Franca declared during the session, "you tell me something". Promptly the therapist replied: "Maybe a fairy tale!"

A delicate clinical fragment, one of the many that punctuate *Psychoanalytic Psychotherapy Between Identity and Change*, a book skilfully edited and introduced by Luigia Cresti and Isabella Lapi, which brings together essays by the same editors together with colleagues from the Associazione Fiorentina di Psicoterapia Psicoanalitica (AFPP): Antonio Suman, Esmeralda Di Mauro, Giulia Mercuriali, Corrado D'Agostini, Alfredina Fiori, Cristina Pratesi, Stefania Pampaloni, Cristina Diana Canzio, enriched by the Foreword by Rosa Romano Toscani.

Tell me a story, tell me a fairy tale, tell me... it is a taste of childhood, like bread with oil or with jam and butter. On the one hand, the many possible examples referring to the "psychotherapist at work" well exemplify one of the fundamental training objectives of the association as the figure of an authentic psychotherapist – open, capable of being in contact with the patient, "malleable" and at the same time rigorous in continually reflecting on technique and the clinic; on the other hand, they shed light on the great changes that psychoanalytic psychotherapy must deal with today, in facing new pathologies for which multiple and different intervention strategies are necessary. Moreover, even Christopher Bollas (2018) warns how, in the age of bewilderment, the depth of the internal world and the sense of being a subject, the ability to tolerate psychic pain and process it, rather than expelling it in a blind enactment, are precisely what gets lost. We thus witness peculiar psychic functioning and unusual pathologies such as – just to name a few – deficiencies in the construction and functioning of identity and symbolic capacities, pathologies in which psyche and soma are often confused, thought does not organise itself but dissolves into acting out and where repression gives way to dissociation. Extending psychodynamic treatments to this different clinical population thus implies – amid uncertainties and pain, amid unexpected discoveries and trust – also substantial modifications of both theory and technique.

Never obviously reduced to a lame imitation of psychoanalysis, the image of psychotherapy that is affirmed in unison in this unmissable book is that of an open process that adapts to the uniqueness and authenticity of the relationship between therapist and patient in the profound conviction that the patient needs the reality of the psychotherapist's emotions in order to feel the reality of his or her own person; in other words, in order to exist, everyone needs to be "seen" and to be "dreamed".

Founded more than 40 years ago, in 1979, the AFPP has, ever since its birth, endeavoured to define, clarify and make known to the general public the particular aspects of the psychotherapeutic approach. And among the many merits that the association possesses is also that of not being afraid of writing, on the contrary, of having promoted, over the years and without relenting, a serious and helpful effort to divulge contemporary contributions as well as the international debate thanks to *Contrappunto*, the association's scientific journal.

In times of a "liquid society", in the midst of a pandemic that is gripping young and old alike, and with the addition today of the echoes of the winds of war, the present work, which is the result of the study group "Table of Thoughts", made up of the authors together with some other AFPP members, vigorously proposes and reformulates some evergreen questions such as: what does it mean to be a psychoanalytic psychotherapist today?, what changing problems and demands must be answered? At the same time, it proposes new questions: what is the importance of the therapist's personality in conducting therapy?, and, last but not least, how to integrate fidelity to proven practices and theories with the variants – slight infidelities – to which the therapist's creativity sometimes resorts in order to meet patients and support them in the symbolic representation of their own internal worlds.

In this sense, Dina Vallino (2021) has often posed the question of how to stimulate the imagination, often withered or crushed by fear in young patients, finding the answer in a sort of homeopathic principle of the mind: "cure imagination with imagination", never disdaining, therefore, to bring into play one's own imagination, one's fantasy, one's artistic and cultural aptitudes, expressing herself in the first person, or drawing, or telling stories in the therapy room.

Here then, the Table of Thoughts delivers to the press, to insiders, (but not only) a book with a high narrative tone and a decisive, sharp, open gaze, towards a future that is not conventional or pre-packaged. A precious, useful and beautiful book, like an ancient Mediterranean garden, "fruitful and delightful". A book that welcomes restlessness, never neglecting the peripheral vision of things; a book that urges one to be vast and to navigate every sea and discover a safe harbour between one wave and another, between impermanence and risk. A book that spurs the creative, innovative reflection of healing methods that do not shy away from the task of sustaining hope and treasuring, like a proud Thumbelina, the crumbs of the arcane bonds that lie behind pain.

Through a careful and lively illustration of some clinical stories, readers will find themselves involved in reflections on the technique of psychoanalytic psychotherapy, ranging from a poignant tactile language to a musical one, up to "imaginative conjectures", to clinging glances as well as dreams as a possible stage, a pathway where the therapist – also thanks to their own dreams, and the incursion into other areas of knowledge such as art, myth, literature – becomes a bridge that allows the passage between bodily reality and psyche, amplifying the patients' own understanding. All this always with the attention turned towards the communicative processes underlying treatment.

Between the pages flow narratives of children, teenagers, adults. There is Emma with her Little Red Riding Hood, Elena locked in her reserve, Antonio caught up in the ideals of perfection, Adriana frozen in her feelings; there is Fiona, there are the tears in Paolo's eyes and the gazes turned to the empty mirror by Alina, there are Anita, Anna, Carolina, and again Rosa, Marta, and Giulia, who in the sweetness of the therapist finally finds "the right warm breast".

The language chosen for the narrative reflects the emotional climate in which psychotherapy takes place. It resounds with poetry – a corporeal, cellular language, as the poet Chandra Candiani (2018) defines it. Because after all, the subversive power of poetic language is precisely that of saying what cannot be said, of making the unimaginable imaginable, of giving livability to the whirlpool of "thoughts in search of a thinker".

Lucid and impassioned, indeed poetic stories intertwined with essential conceptualizations of the founders of psychoanalysis, (such as Sigmund Freud, Melanie Klein, Sandor Ferenczi, Michael Balint, Wilfred Bion, Donald Winnicott, Esther Bick etc.), as well as of the most authoritative contemporary psychoanalysts: Otto Kernberg, Stefano Bolognini, Philip Bromberg, Antonino Ferro, Ralph Greenson, Clara Mucci, Allan Shore, the clinicians of the Boston Change Process Group and many others.

The theoretical framework is, therefore, strong and solid, and yet, in the various essays, it never loses that pleasant, homelike tone – which Walter Benjamin would not have hesitated to define as "azure" (2006) – everything is sustained by the affection and the gratitude towards the Masters with whom the Association has dealt and grown since its beginnings, from Donald Meltzer and Martha Harris, to Franco and Gina Mori, Adolfo Pazzagli, Giovanni Hautmann, Francisco Palacio Espasa and Anne Alvarez.

Now, on closing the book and paraphrasing the title of Antonio Suman's fine essay "And the door closes", the space of the heart remains palpitating, the liveliness of the analysis room remains, where one can let oneself go, without fear (or, not infrequently, together with fear) and where, in Winnicott's terms, one learns to "be alone in the presence of someone".

"It's nice to come here!", little Clara exclaims, almost in repartee, as she experiments like a scientist in a session. And philosophically, she concludes: "In this silence, thoughts are released."

Yes, because in the proximity, in the assonance between poetry and therapeutic work, "honest" silence, as Chandra Candiani writes, "is a living thing". And above all, as the poet summarises, reversing Clara's words: "Silence sows. Words reap."

References

Benjamin, W. (2006). *Berlin Childhood around 1900*. Cambridge, MA: Harvard University Press.

Bollas, C. (2018). *Meaning and Melancholia: The Age of Bewilderment*. London: Routledge.

Candiani, L.C. (2018). *Il silenzio è cosa viva*. Turin: Einaudi.

Vallino, D. (2021). *Raccontami una storia*. Milan: Mimesis.

Introduction

Luigia Cresti and Isabella Lapi

What does it mean to be a psychoanalytic psychotherapist today? What kind of problems and demands are we called upon to respond to? How are the psychoanalytic theoretical assumptions underlying our training translated into our practice? How do we integrate fidelity to them with the small "betrayals" to which the therapist's creativity must sometimes resort? And what are the elective technical tools we use? How important is the therapist's personality in conducting treatment?

These questions have accompanied us since the early 1980s, weaving themselves into a more general question of identity that we have attempted to answer throughout our training and experiential journey.

Our reflection on these themes was originally driven by the need to define our identity as psychotherapists and the theoretical-clinical model that guided our work. In Chapter 1, we will briefly illustrate the historical path that has crossed the research carried out in the Associazione Fiorentina di Psicoterapia Psicoanalitica (AFPP). aimed at focusing on the specific and peculiar features that properly connote a psychotherapy as psychoanalytic. In our associative course of study and research on clinical experience, we have always tried to elaborate a flexible technical model of conduct, while respecting a sufficiently rigorous setting, and one that is not reduced to an imitation of psychoanalysis; we have given importance to knowing how to be with the patient in a spontaneous way, appealing to our authenticity and favouring relational aspects; we have also chosen to adopt greater flexibility in the adjustment of the setting in particular situations.

Today, we are faced with important changes in psychic pathology and therapeutic demand, which often entail, in both private and public practice, modifications of settings and unusual technical choices, which raise the need to rethink the practice of psychoanalytic psychotherapy and redefine it in relation to the changed context, while maintaining its original theoretical grounds and its profoundly transformative aims.

The current work of the study group, known as the "Table of Thoughts", is in this vein, recovering points of reflection already proposed in the past in the AFPP and then at the Italian Section of the European Federation for

DOI: 10.4324/9781032673721-1

Psychoanalytic Psychotherapy (EFPP). It was precisely on the occasion of the 1st SIEFPP National Meeting in 2014, held in Rome, that a paper was presented, entitled "La psicoterapia psicoanalitica oggi: delimitazioni, fattori terapeutici, nuove prospettive" [Psychoanalytic psychotherapy today: delimitations, therapeutic factors, new perspectives] (Cresti and Suman, 2014), which constituted an outline later reworked and enriched together in the work of the Table. A focal point of that report was the non-interpretive therapeutic factors, first and foremost, the containing functions of the therapeutic *enveloppe*; other related aspects (such as the increased attention to the body, the use of unusual interventions, such as *Interpret Actions*) were then the subject of further in-depth study in the context of the Table of Thoughts, in which the constant reference to the participants' professional clinical experience was central.

The study group consisted of Luigia Cresti, Isabella Lapi, Cristina Pratesi, as well as Cristina Canzio, Esmeralda Di Mauro, Alfredina Fiori, Elisa Larini, Giulia Mercuriali, Stefania Pampaloni, and Antonio Suman; an interesting contribution was subsequently made by Corrado D'Agostini.

The group's working methodology consisted of monthly meetings over the course of two years, in which clinical and theoretical materials relating to various focuses were presented. The participants took turns to write reports that formed the thread of the meetings, and then to draft a final report. In our view, the presentation of the reports of the meetings took on an important significance, as they indicated the shaping of the thoughts of the group.

This group sharing of clinical experiences, and the resulting thoughts, correspond to one of the basic principles underlying the founding of the AFPP and its training: the life of our association has always been animated by constant confrontation and discussion; peer-to-peer exchange has been privileged in our cultural activity and is the basis of our research method, in the conviction that this promotes the growth of all members.

As our in-depth study continued and the group's thinking was built up, the idea of sharing it with colleagues on an increasingly broader basis began to emerge: first, in seminars open to psychotherapists from other associations[1] and then with this book.

Once the roundtable meetings were over, the work continued with in-depth discussion among the members, individually or in small groups; these contributions, however, despite their diversity, were deeply shared among us in a unified manner.

Writing represented a further development of thought: by putting them down on paper, our thoughts were becoming sharper and richer and, by association, more thoughts emerged, always with the desire to compare them with the ideas of other colleagues and the positions of various authors, drawing on the rich mine of thoughts that is psychoanalytic theory.

The various chapters touch on the themes on which the group's attention has focused: Chapter 1 ("Psychoanalytic psychotherapy between identity and change") presents a brief historical survey from the 1980s to the present day on the evolution of the models and technique of psychoanalytic psychotherapy in its relationship with psychoanalysis, following the development of the debate within the AFPP. Ample space has been given to our roots, which represent a solid and secure starting point, exemplifying and in some ways anticipating the debate that has developed over the years around the identity of psychoanalytic psychotherapy. When we began, other scientific societies of psychoanalytic psychotherapy were also appearing on the Italian scene and the dominant theme was its differentiation from psychoanalysis, at first seen in the concrete aspects of the setting (reduced number of weekly sessions, the use of face-to-face setting, the focusing of therapeutic objectives, etc.). then, little by little, also in its technical aspects (Brignone et al., 1998). At that time, it was necessary to define oneself, even by difference, to feel oneself as a protagonist and not as "children of a lesser God". Much time has passed; today the scene is changing and is moving in the direction of thinking about a continuum between psychoanalysis and psychoanalytic psychotherapy, considered as part of the larger family of psychodynamic psychotherapy, and overcoming what is now widely called the "narcissism of small differences". The work we present starts, therefore, from history and then explores the new, the changes of today. The strong and disorienting changes in what Bollas (2018) has called "the age of bewilderment" – in which what gets lost is precisely the depth of the internal world and the sense of being a subject, the ability to tolerate psychic pain and process it, rather than expelling it in a blind enactment – lead to new psychic functioning and new pathologies, such as deficiencies in the construction and functioning of identity and symbolic capacities (see Chapter 7, "Adaptations of technique in the psychotherapy of borderline patients" and Chapter 6, "Patients unable to dream"). Psychotherapy is an important observation point for this bewilderment that affects everyone: changes are brought into our rooms in a strong way by the patients, necessitating new readings of clinical phenomena and the use of therapeutic functions that are quite different from our classic interpretative tools. The space within which the therapist must move in order to best identify and deal with the multiplicity of patients' needs is vast and varied; in it the therapist will have to move, following different paths, separate or intersecting, depending on the objectives to be achieved, relying on the compass offered by psychoanalytic tools. Among these, in our opinion, the tools pertaining to the non-interpretive therapeutic factors must be valued and used to the greatest extent: the relationship, first of all, composed of looking and listening to, in order to offer visual and sound containment (see Chapter 2, "Non-interpretive therapeutic factors: the containing functions in the therapeutic relationship"); the recognition of the body, both of the patient and of the therapist, as a vehicle of important meanings and messages. In fact, bodily components are inevitably present in the therapeutic relationship; recognizing them allows us to pay attention to the non-verbal messages that the patient conveys to us, to the bodily sensations experienced by the therapist, as indicators of significant, non-verbal aspects that the patient projects onto us; within this theme we also wanted to address the interesting and little-explored topic of the implications connected to the therapist's pregnancy. And then the therapist's own actions (see Chapter 4, "Gestures that touch, actions that heal"). now recognized in their communicative value, sometimes alternative to – and more effective than – verbal communication; the new territories that open up for the therapist to meet the patient, such as his/her own dreams, which in our relational perspective we prefer not to call countertransference (see Chapter 5, "New territories for the patient: the therapist's dreams" and, for example, the section "The therapist's dreams in supervision"); the enhancement of the patients' artistic expression, which offers them a way to access the symbolic representation of the internal world (see Chapter 8, "Psychotherapy and artistic expression"). Going through the various chapters, we wanted to bring out the figure of a psychotherapist who is authentic, open, capable of always being in contact with the patient, "malleable"[2] and at the same time rigorous in continually reflecting on technique and the clinic. In fact, all the chapters contain numerous clinical illustrations taken from the psychotherapy of children, adolescents and adults, which show the above-mentioned issues in real life.

This choice is consistent with the methodological principle underlying our training and research, as we have also learnt from Infant Observation training: the formulation of hypotheses, or "imaginative conjectures", as new ideas and operational proposals can only arise from the careful observation and recording of clinical data.

In the book, we also report on some particular experiences that enabled us not to lose contact with patients during the periods of distance imposed by the COVID-19 pandemic and the protection measures (see Chapter 9, "'Leading our caravans to the West': psychotherapy at a distance" and "The musicality of the voice in telephone consultations" (AFPP, 2021), the latter, the result of the experience of the voluntary and free consultations carried out in the listening service initiated by the AFPP during the pandemic[3]), which allowed us to better understand some therapeutic functions by adding new tools to our toolbox.

The book closes with Chapter 10 ("... And the door closes: concluding reflections") that encourages reflection on the therapist's thoughts after the patient's session has ended; generally little considered, the time spent taking notes, reflecting or analysing one's countertransference is actually part of the therapeutic process and helps the therapist to become more aware and to resolve possible impasses.

The rapid social, cultural and technological changes in today's world, which have such an impact on the formation of the person and his or her mental health, impose themselves not only on the psychotherapeutic approach but also on all the disciplines that in various ways deal with mankind, including moral philosophy and ethics.

This is the message that runs throughout our book and that we want to convey to colleagues who will read and reflect with us. The picture of psychotherapy that we have in mind is that of a very open process that adapts to the uniqueness and authenticity of the relationship that develops between therapist and patient; it will be different each time, each time it will teach something to both partners; it will always be a different journey amid uncertainties and pain, new discoveries and trust. To face it, the therapist will need the well-equipped baggage of psychoanalytic theory, which continues to provide fundamental and profound tools to be used in an agile and flexible manner.

Our initial questions will not be fully answered in the book: fundamentally, if we think about it, they do not have to be, because the vitality of a person, a theory, a technique lies in continuous change and adaptation; a rigid theory is the opposite of thinking.

Just as, at the end of the session, the therapist closes the door of the room behind the patient but continues thinking about him/her, we hope that our research journey will continue over time … because, after all, we know that the beauty of the journey is the path one takes, rather than reaching the destination!

Notes

1 Two seminars were organised involving SIPP (Società Italiana di Psicoterapia Psicoanalitica), IIPG (Istituto Italiano di Psicoanalisi di Gruppo) and CSMH-AMHPPIA (Centro Studi Martha Harris), both centred on psychoanalytic psychotherapy today: in 2020, "New paths, new identities?" and in 2021, "Insights and new perspectives".
2 We use this term in a technical sense, borrowing it from the research of Vacheret (2001) and Roussillon (2020).
3 An association, even if scientific and aimed at psychotherapy, is not detached but rather immersed in the world, breathing and living together with the context in which it operates. The profound, real and phantasmal unease created by the pandemic did not leave us indifferent and, responding to the so-called social vocation of psychoanalysis, we moved to offer our professionalism free of charge. This experience is collected in the book *Prendersi cura nell'emergenza* [Caring in an Emergency] (AFPP, 2021). Another offer of voluntary help from AFPP members and students, together with other psychoanalytic associations, is currently being made to refugees from the Ukraine.

References

AFPP (2021). *Prendersi cura nell'emergenza*. Florence: Tassinari.
Bollas, C. (2018). *Meaning and Melancholia: The Age of Bewilderment*. London: Routledge.
Brignone, A., D'Agostini, C., Fiorentini, N., Lumachi, A., Mori, L., Puccetti, F., Russo, S., Scarpellini, L., Trapani, G., and Tubi, V. (1998). Possibilità di un lavoro psicoanalitico nelle psicoterapie monosettimanali. In M. Gino and R. Romano Toscani (eds), *Ritmo e setting*. Rome: Borla.
Cresti, L. and Suman, A. (2014). La psicoterapia psicoanalitica oggi: delimitazioni, fattori terapeutici, nuove prospettive (unpublished text).
Roussillon, R. (2020). Nuovi paradigmi per le pratiche cliniche (unpublished text).
Vacheret, C. (2001). Il Gruppo e l'oggetto intermedio: il photolangage nel lavoro clinico. *Contrappunto*, 28: 21–35.

Chapter 1

Identity and change

Luigia Cresti and Antonio Suman

New paradigms for new scenarios

Today, psychotherapists are confronted with major social, cultural and economic changes, which call for a rethink of the practice of psychoanalytic psychotherapy and defining it more clearly in relation to the changed context, while retaining its original theoretical grounding and its profoundly transformative aims.

Under the pressure of environmental and social changes, psychic distress is also taking on different contours and characteristics; one need only think of certain phenomena that characterize today's social and psychological scenarios, such as the instability of families and the precarious or conflictual couple, and parental relationships in which children are often involved, with obvious consequences on the structuring of their personalities. The quality of relational exchanges is also changing: through social media, as opportunities for encounters have multiplied, at the expense, however, of the depth of relationships, which are thus being superficialized, with the loss of meta-social guarantees.[1] Such superficialization also applies to the current modes of transmission and acquisition of information, which pass through the visual and are therefore mediated by the immediateness and simultaneity of the inputs. More generally, it seems that identity formation processes, the transmission of transgenerational fantasies, and unconscious identifications are brought into play. The greater freedom of thought and culture available to adolescents and young adults, although positive, also produces more anxiety because the developmental process becomes more fluid. In the delicate transition from adolescence to adulthood, the rituals that existed in the past and are still practised in more primitive cultures, have given way to much longer, more complex and also more uncertain paths. There is no longer a clear distinction between male and female gender, a wider freedom of choice is common, but this also entails greater difficulty in finding one's own path adapted to personal qualities and expectations; even male and female sexual roles, active and passive, are almost interchangeable: proof of this is the phenomenon, which we have observed in our clinical work, of a readiness among young people to experience homosexual – and heterosexual – relationships indistinctly.

DOI: 10.4324/9781032673721-2

Psychoanalytic psychotherapy today has to deal with these changes, coping with new pathologies that require new intervention strategies; pathologies in which psyche soma are confused, and thinking does not organize itself but dissolves in acting out, and repression gives way to dissociation (McWilliams, 2019). Extending psychodynamic treatments to this diverse clinical population implies substantial modifications in both theory and technique. There is no doubt, however, that for a large part of the symptomatology presented by today's patients, it is not enough to simply interpret the unconscious repressed contents, according to a psychoanalytic classical model, but pinpointing and developing other interventions are required.

In order to address such complex issues that differ from the disorders traditionally addressed by psychoanalysis, psychotherapeutic treatments can make use of research developed in related fields, foremost neuroscience, which studies individual psychic functions and their localization in the central and peripheral nervous system. This broadening of the contributions of the knowledge that can be integrated into treatments partly modifies the techniques of psychoanalytic psychotherapy, which today we should perhaps more appropriately call "psychodynamic psychotherapy", underlining this diversity of research and development. In short, the problem is how to adapt psychotherapeutic technique, modulating it in a synthesis between continuity and innovation.

The new social, psychological and clinical scenarios pose a challenge that we now have to deal with in our daily practice, which requires the ability to tolerate doubts, uncertainties, and flexibly adapt possible intervention strategies. A common problem, for example, is how to conduct psychoanalytic psychotherapy treatment when only once a week or even fortnightly attendance is possible, or what the increasingly frequent use of online sessions entails, not least because of the pandemic situation. It is also a challenging task to maintain a psychodynamic setting in situations of brief or time-limited psychotherapeutic interventions.

Such questions require the therapist to continually adapt known mental and operational models to new situations, where it sometimes seems difficult to preserve the correct psychodynamic procedure (see Box 1.1).

Box 1.1 The current psychopathological scenario

Underlying the symptoms presented by today's patients there are increasingly frequent problems linked to strong psychological components, such as anxiety disorders, mood disorders and personality organization difficulties. These conditions have a numerical prevalence over those of psychiatric relevance, which are characterized by a significant genetic component, such as schizophrenia, bipolar disorders, and obsessive-compulsive disorders.

Anxiety disorders and panic attacks are almost ubiquitous in current psychopathological contexts and result, in 50 per cent of cases, in social phobia and agoraphobia. They are mainly triggered by fantasies of being unable to escape or of not having a way back home (see, for example, the inability to drive on the motorway). There is a sense of loss of real or imaginary attachment figures resulting in fantasies of physical collapse or of going mad. Underlying these phenomena, it is possible to discern the lack of valid identification figures. Among mood disorders, depressions linked to feelings of inadequacy and shame are more frequent than those related to guilt.

Borderline personality organizations and syndromes that lack verbalization and symbolization are increasing; body-centred pathologies that express themselves through, for example, eating disorders, self-inflicted injuries and psychosomatic disorders are also frequent. For years, problems have arisen from drug addiction with old and new drugs, alcohol, gambling or new addictions such as those related to the Web.

Rather than the attainment of pleasure, these behaviours are not infrequently oriented towards the manipulation of emotional states, such as the "high", which is not necessarily a pleasurable state per se, but rather a manipulation of the state of mind, a way of avoiding emotions that cannot be controlled and that frighten many adolescents and young adults.

Underlying various symptoms are very often problems which refer originally to critical issues in the attachment process and the resulting difficulties in integrating the personality. Events therefore arise that are not mentalized but remain anchored in the body and are expressed through it, thus remaining outside the verbal register. Traumas that affect children in the pre-verbal period emerge significantly, and although they cannot be put into words, they are no less laden with pathogenic consequences, in the same way as non-verbalized traumas that occur later in life, which can be associated with memory disorders and re-emerge in a repetitive way through acting out or enactment.

It is precisely for this reason that the subject of psychic traumas and their psycho-material consequences has become an area of research that increasingly has been developing.

The psychological and social malaise was also heightened by the fear triggered by the COVID-19 pandemic and the isolation imposed by the norms that regulated everyday life. The closeness in enclosed spaces activated ambivalent feelings between desire and danger and became a source of uneasiness and anxiety. This led to more or less severe depressive responses, including an increase in suicidal ideation. The numbers of adolescents who turned to the Child Neuropsychiatry Service of the Bambino Gesù Hospital in Rome in 2021 after having attempted suicide increased from 36 per cent to 63 per cent.

Our research path to the current vision

The intention is to carry out an investigation to focus and define more clearly the peculiar aspects of the psychotherapeutic approach, verifying its appropriateness and legitimacy, and this has been central in the history of the Florentine Association of Psychoanalytic Psychotherapy (AFPP) since its founding in 1979. At its basis, as the association's founding statute states, there was the aim of:

fostering an in-depth ability to conduct the therapeutic relationship by following an organic program that took into account clinical activity, specific theoretical acquisitions and emotional experiences connected to psychotherapeutic work and group activities ... The theory to be constantly referred to is the psychoanalytic one as a fundamental tool for understanding both intrapsychic reality and the relationship.

(Suman, 1987)

But even then, we felt that the problem of transferring the theoretical knowledge we had acquired, together with the experience of our own analysis, to an operational activity that developed in different contexts – for example, in institutions – and addressed patients with multiple forms of discomfort and new demands (e.g., psychotic children and adults, cases of social maladjustment, patients with psychosomatic suffering, etc.) remained open. We believe that similar paths to ours have also marked the growth of other Italian psychotherapy associations and have similarly accompanied the ongoing debate within the European Federation for Psychoanalytic Psychotherapy (EFPP), of which we are members.[2]

Therefore, in outlining here the decades-long reflection developed within the AFPP, aimed at focusing on which specific aspects characterize psychoanalytic psychotherapy and what are its technical cornerstones, we do not intend to offer a self-referential account from a narrow local perspective, but rather to suggest topics for discussion, in-depth analysis and comparison with colleagues from other associations and training schools, even those who are geographically distant.

Our research has been stimulated over the past decades not only by the numerous individual and group supervision experiences we have all had in the course of our training, but above all by the continual comparison with clinically and scientifically important figures, both nationally and internationally, during the numerous seminars we have organized (we would just like to mention D. Meltzer, M. Harris, A. Alvarez, F. Palacio-Espasa and, closer to us, Gina and Franco Mori, G. Hautmann, and A. Pazzagli). We are grateful to them all for their help in defining the main parameters that characterize psychotherapy as psychoanalytic. Even though their indications and clarifications date back decades, they have nonetheless shaped the fundamental structures of our thinking.

For our part, we were well aware from the outset that the reference to psychoanalytic theory and its basic technical instruments was indispensable, but in the face of the variety of curative demands and the changing pathology and socio-economic-cultural reality, we wanted to develop a technical model of therapeutic conduct that was flexible and did not simply imitate psychoanalysis, although it used its basic theoretical and technical assumptions. A valuable opportunity for reflection and enrichment was provided by the interviews with our masters, which were regularly published between 1987 and 1992 in *Contrappunto*, the scientific journal of our association. We asked them questions about the implications of a reduced frequency of sessions (typical of psychotherapy), about the use and interpretation of transference and counter-transference,[3] about the appropriateness of analyzing patients' conscious expectations of psychotherapy, about considering evaluative and/or predictive aspects, etc. The articulate and stimulating answers of our interlocutors constituted an important track along this path to define more clearly the specificity of psychoanalytic psychotherapy. In parallel with this learning experience, self-managed study-groups were formed within the AFPP, which often resulted in local seminars or contributions to national and international seminars.

We propose here, in brief, some of the basic ideas that have developed over the years within our association, according to the advice of our teachers:

- D. Meltzer explained that in order to do psychoanalytic psychotherapy, it is essential to create a setting in which a transference relationship can develop; it is precisely the establishment of this relationship that makes a process "psychoanalytic". It can also be initiated regardless of the number of sessions. Transference interpretation is a constituent element of both psychoanalysis and psychoanalytic psychotherapy.

- This theme was expanded by F. Palacio-Espasa, who pointed out how the type of transference varies according to the setting one decides to establish, and the process that will be determined depends on this choice. Thus, the choice of a setting must be consequent to the preliminary assessment of the patient and the diagnostic study of the organization of his/her personality. In his opinion, attention to symptoms is crucial, since they are not "secondary epiphenomena" – as they have often been considered by traditional psychoanalysis – but are instead deep expressions of the patient's conflicting psychic internal states and object relations. Symptomatic changes are a goal to be pursued, as they indicate changes in the internal structure. Psychotherapy must therefore tend towards the elimination or alleviation of symptoms.

- Pazzagli's model, also appeared to us extremely lucid and precise: according to it, psychoanalytically-oriented psychotherapy has three fundamental parameters:direct, explicit and sought-after purpose of treatment … specific interest in symptoms and behaviour, understood, however, not only as external manifestations but as internal phenomena, as ideas and emotions. A symptom can acquire a new meaning within the therapeutic relationship, which allows it to be metabolized, making it thinkable and comprehensible. Psychoanalytic psychotherapy starts with the symptoms, but gradually widens the scope of what lies behind them. From this premise derives the need to accept the value of reality from the outset. This is also reflected in the choice of the specific setting for psychotherapy, which, unlike psychoanalysis, is characterized by face-to-face therapy, a reduced number of weekly sessions and often a more limited duration of time. Like Palacio-Espasa, therefore, Pazzagli also supported the usefulness of the preliminary assessment, the importance of paying attention to symptoms, and above all, the consideration that "a different setting characterizes a different type of relationship".

The fundamental difference between the psychotherapeutic process and the psychoanalytic process, according to Pazzagli, can be formulated as follows: Psychotherapy starts from the real towards the mental by including it more and more, and psychoanalysis starts from the limit of the un-mentalized by making it mental and tending towards the real. In the same way, with respect to the nature of the object, it can be said that psychotherapy, through sensory control, starts from the real object but goes towards the meanings of the archaic object; psychoanalysis starts from the archaic object and its precursors but sees how the archaic object is still real, and therefore goes in the opposite direction.

Both, psychotherapy and psychoanalysis, are therefore, "North Stars" for each other; there is no problem of hierarchy but there are differences: psychotherapy has its own different setting and must be aware of its own value. The psychotherapist's training must also follow its own original path, as must supervision.

At that time, the idea of a psychoanalytic psychotherapy that has its own setting, that deals with healing, that considers the level of reality in order to introduce the symbolic level, that makes use of various therapeutic instruments including transference interpretations, was emerging in our group: a psychoanalytic psychotherapy that uses psychoanalytic theory but with its own specificity of goals, technique and training.

Psychotherapy and psychoanalysis: what is their relationship?

Along the path of reflection and research that we have pursued over these years, we too have discussed the problem of the differences, especially on a technical level, between psychoanalytic psychotherapy and psychoanalysis. We know that this debate has spanned the history of the last century in the European and American cultural context and has perhaps not yet led to entirely definitive answers.[4] It is not our intention here to go into the vexed historical course of the question of the differences between psychoanalytic psychotherapy and psychoanalysis. We will limit ourselves, as far as the more recent debate in Europe is concerned, to citing a collected text (Frisch, Hinshelwood and Gauthier, 2001) by the EFPP that opens with a Foreword by R. Wallerstein, who defines psychoanalytic psychotherapy as "a set of concepts and techniques based on psychoanalytic theory, but adapted to the different clinical needs of those patients who are not considered suitable for the rigidity of psychoanalysis proper, within a classical psychoanalytic understanding". With regard to the question of whether psychoanalytic psychotherapy is the "legitimate or illegitimate heir of psychoanalysis", he calls for a rethink on the numerous unanswered questions, proposing that future studies and reflections focus on the neutral problem of the nature and principles of psychic change. Wallerstein (2001) adds that "throughout the psychoanalytic world, shared certainties about the strict distinctions between psychoanalysis and psychoanalytic psychotherapy no longer exist".

The boundaries that demarcated psychoanalytic psychotherapy and psychoanalysis are now blurred and constantly shifting, depending on one's starting position or theoretical predilections.

As for the discussion in Italy, historically there have been alternating tendencies to differentiate or associate psychotherapy and psychoanalysis together (Turillazzi, 1979), in particular, during the 1970s and 1980s, a debate on this issue flared up in Italy, with opposing opinions and positions, also because the nascent psychotherapy associations were looking for their own definition, at the same time as different models were spreading, with reference both to psychoanalysis and other cultural orientations (e.g., relational systemic and cognitive-behavioural). Among other things, the possibility of introducing psychoanalytic psychotherapy, with appropriate adjustments, into public institutions was discussed.

More recently, we have the impression that there is a tendency to consider the two approaches – the strictly psychoanalytic and the psychotherapeutic one – as being placed along a continuum; there are probably times when psychoanalysis works in a psychotherapeutic sense and psychotherapy works in a psychoanalytic sense; the paths of reflection on the aims of each type of intervention and the instruments to pursue them often seem to converge.

From the point of view of technique, we can think, in brief, that psychoanalysis and psychoanalytic psychotherapy are approaching each other, particularly with regard to certain aspects:

• The first important point is the *purpose of therapy*. In an article, the psychoanalyst M. Ponsi (2012) argued:

Although bringing the unconscious to consciousness remains, especially in the general public, the goal of analysis, it cannot be said that this goal is shared by psychoanalysts today ... In contemporary, post-classical psychoanalytic schools, the priority given to the cognitive goal has diminished ... For the purposes of change, rather than calling into question the unconscious-consciousness transition, attention is paid to the analytic relationship, the transference-countertransference dynamics and the therapeutic alliance ... Insight has been taken off the pedestal and the fundamental importance of the relationship for therapeutic change has been brought to the fore.

This position coincides with the conviction, which has always underpinned the psychotherapeutic approach, that our work – defined by some as "more democratic and aimed at a healthy realism" (Suman and Brignone, 2001) – should first and foremost have a specifically curative task and that this can be achieved mainly through the emotional relationship with the therapist as a person.

- Another crucially important point is, in our opinion, that of the *therapeutic factors*; in this respect, too, we have noted in recent years the existence of numerous points of convergence, whereby the research paths and technical choices made simultaneously in the psychoanalytic and psychotherapeutic spheres tend to come closer together.

Some psychoanalysts question whether the classical device is unsuitable for some patients and think that the traditional technique should therefore be revised: a leading exponent of this view is A.M. Niccolò, who has argued on several occasions (2003; 2019) that interpretation is not "the only arrow in the analyst's quiver", that one must "pay attention to the existence of different levels of symbolization in patients", and that "no interpretation is effective because of its truth, but because of the affectivity it conveys, which makes the truth comprehensible".

Other authors (Bromberg, 1998; Mucci, 2020) also argue that verbal interpretation has no effect with "difficult" patients; rather, it is necessary to work with an empathic closeness that encompasses their actions inside and outside the setting (Bolognini, 2018), providing a mirror and a somatic rêverie that differs from the "opaque" withdrawal of their caregivers. These positions converge, moreover, with what G.O. Gabbard and D. Westen (2003) and the clinicians of the Boston Change Process Group (2010) had already argued; the idea that unites them is that the meaning given to interpretation should be reviewed: in order to promote therapeutic change, "something more" is needed (*something more than interpretation*). That is, those "moments of encounter" between patient and therapist in the intersubjective relational field, which can activate new ways of being with others.

We would like to add that, even in the context of our reflection on what the salient elements of psychotherapeutic intervention are, these issues have been repeatedly discussed and addressed within the AFPP and brought to the attention of colleagues since 2011. We will limit ourselves here to mentioning a paper we presented at the SIEFPP National Meeting held in Rome in 2014, in which the importance was recalled of reflecting on non-interpretative therapeutic factors, which can work "alongside" or "instead of" classical technical instruments or that in any case are intertwined with them. The basic question posed was: what is it in the therapeutic relationship that heals, besides interpretation? Consequently, the multiple "containing" aspects of the therapeutic framework were examined and, alongside this, the importance of the overall depth of the relationship was emphasized, including the sense of the therapist's own personality that is conveyed by the therapist to the patient; hence the need to explore more deeply the complex links between the intrapsychic and the intersubjective.

In short, at this point, we should say that certain opposing positions, tinged with antagonism, that prevailed in the past no longer seem appropriate nowadays and perhaps the time has come for a more fruitful comparison and integration between the two types of approach. A vision of this kind was also suggested by S. Bolognini (2018), who stated that "the times when psychoanalytic psychotherapy seemed to be a by-product of psychoanalysis are long gone; the former has shown the great merit of recognizing the necessary adaptation to changing needs".

However, this does not mean that the model of psychotherapeutic intervention is interchangeable with the model of psychoanalysis; in fact, in psychotherapeutic practice, we often refrain from using certain theoretical and technical conceptualizations typical of classical psychoanalysis outright.

Summarizing our point of view on the issues raised so far, it is our opinion that psychoanalytic psychotherapy, on the one hand, cannot disregard certain central assumptions of psychoanalysis, which we consider to be the basis of both approaches, such as:

- The interest in the exploration of the individual's internal world and dream-life.
- The offer of a relational space, as a place where inner reality can express itself; through empathic listening. The therapist must make his or her thinking presence felt in the emotional relationship with the patient, so as to foster growth in him or her through the experience of the relationship.
- The therapeutic process must then lead to growth through insight, so that the patient gradually comes into contact with the emotions related to himself/herself, to the psychotherapy and to the therapist.
- Hence the importance of paying attention to the transference and counter-transference dynamics, in the sense that the therapist has to maintain the possibility of a transferential reading of the material produced by the patient and analyze his or her own emotional (and also bodily) responses.
- The psychotherapist must engage in the establishment and maintenance of a clearly defined treatment device, recognizing the fundamental value of the setting.

A prerequisite of our work is to have confidence in the transformative effect of interpretation, aimed at promoting insight.

On the other hand, we have seen how the complex changes in today's society and psychopathology pose new problems for the clinic and new challenges to the technique, making diversified and flexible settings necessary, without abandoning or excessively diluting the theoretical matrix of reference. The focus from the traditional concepts of neutrality or abstinence has shifted to other typically relational concepts, such as containment, interaction, or enactment.

From these considerations derive certain specificities that characterize the psychotherapeutic approach in a particular way:

- The therapeutic aim, which considers symptoms to be important and requires a preliminary assessment and diagnostic profile, does not mean, however, that the therapy is exclusively symptomatic, but it must be a therapy that "cares", and promotes reflective thinking, a sense of security, contact with emotions, integration between the various parts of the personality; a therapy capable of activating the developmental processes that have stalled, or never started, in individuals with disorders related to early blocks in the body-psyche development.
- A greater consideration of the external reality and environmental context; the psychotherapist presents himself/herself more as a real object, also as a consequence of the face-to-face mode of encounter.
- In psychotherapy, there is a greater appreciation of the non-interpretive therapeutic factors, particularly the "containing" and intersubjective ones. Our attention has, in fact, focused, above all, on the significance of the containing function of the therapeutic relationship, in its many facets. Equally important to us is the inter-subjective dimension, i.e., attention to the quality of being together, of emotional contact, to the overall depth of the relationship, and also to the sense of his/her own personality that the therapist conveys to the patient.[5]
- In terms of technique, the use of transference and countertransference interpretations is more "measured" in psychotherapy; interpretations focus heavily on desires, fears and extra-transferential conflicts.

Other aspects that we feel deserve specific consideration in psychotherapeutic practice are:

- Particular attention is paid to communication that is not only verbal but also comes from other extra-verbal communication channels. Hence the recognition of the significant role that the body can play in the therapeutic relationship: that of the patient, first of all, but also that of the therapist (this theme will be addressed in Chapter 3).
- A greater willingness to accept the communicative value of the patient's "acts" and sometimes legitimize the therapist's use of "actions" (as will be illustrated in Chapter 4).

We would like to add, however, that our work here does not have a defining intent, but merely tends to propose a guideline and stimulate research that will have to be further revised and updated: at a time in history when family, environmental and socio-cultural conditions are constantly evolving, we too should be prepared to change our technique and revise our objectives.

Peculiarities of psychotherapy training: Infant Observation

Let us now take up Pazzagli's suggestion that psychotherapist training should follow its own original path. In this regard, in our experiential and clinical journey we have become convinced that the Infant Observation model, according to Esther Bick – a central teaching subject in the AFPP training – is a fundamental tool for the basic training in a psychodynamic perspective and thus an indispensable prerequisite for psychotherapists, also for those who carry out psychotherapeutic work with adults. G. Ferrara Mori, quoting Meltzer, defined it as:

> a unique and original method that requires from the observer a conscious and unconscious understanding of what is being observed, a seeing with the eyes outwards and inwards, a combination that makes an observation valid as a set of psychoanalytic facts on which one can think.
>
> (2001)

A "neutral participant observation" of the relationship between the young child and its family during the first years of life – a fundamental experience in our training – allows us to perceive the constitution of the self and of the primary "object relationships", to better understand non-verbal behaviour and play in children, and their psycho-affective development in the family.

Observational training is also an important premise for the acquisition of a solid psychotherapeutic attitude, through respect for the setting, neutrality, the exercise of accepting the mother's projective identifications and tolerating the primitive anxieties projected by the child; in the psychotherapy of children, but also of adults, it helps us to grasp and to give meaning to body language and recognize the legacy of early experiences in patients. Infant Observation is a method that encourages the development of a receptive sensitivity, the ability to observe without preconceptions and preconceived assumptions, using one's intuition and subjectivity as a means of knowledge. This experience can therefore result in the acquisition of better intervention tools and new ways of understanding the transformative processes inherent in every therapeutic process.

Particularly significant in this respect is the observation that in many long-term family observation experiences, a therapeutic value for the mother-child relationship has unexpectedly emerged; in various observation situations, even though there were no explicit aims of treatment nor interpretative interventions, components were activated in the mother-child-observer relationship, which to a certain extent laid the foundations for a better development of it.[6]

The therapeutic components of the observational process have, moreover, been highlighted by several prominent authors: M. Pérez-Sanchez, G. Polacco Williams, and G. Ferrara Mori (2001), who pointed out that contact with the observer's non-verbal but mental functions, with his/her sustained attention and gaze – the equivalent of listening – enables the child and his or her family to make an initial transformation of their emotional experiences and helps to contain painful experiences rather than evacuate them.[7]

Here, the comparison with the clinical-professional experience of treatment arises spontaneously, in which the therapeutic process is often made possible and activated by precisely those relational factors that can give to the observation an implicit value of support and care; they have to do with the functions of containment in its various meanings (a theme that will be dealt with at length in Chapter 2).

The supervision of a psychoanalytic psychotherapist[8]

The topic of supervision was discussed and explored in depth, starting with our commitment as training teachers in the AFPP Postgraduate School. The result was the identification of some "guiding ideas" consistent with our vision of psychoanalytic psychotherapy: in general, we share L. Grinberg's (1989) position on supervision, considered as "a learning process that occurs both in the student and in the teacher: they become observers of an experience that enriches them both".

An important function of supervision is when the supervisor takes on a position of "participant observer", i.e., of empathetic participation. This aspect has been emphasized, in particular, by R. Greenson (1974), who considers the supervisor's task of stimulating the student's ability to use empathy to be central. The main difficulty for the supervisor is that of integrating the various functions of teaching, attention to empathy and countertransference, and at the same time evaluating the student. With regard to the supervisor's task as "teacher", in our practice, we agree with O. Kernberg's (2003) suggestion to introduce theoretical references linked to clinical work, being careful, however, not to burden the supervisee's mind with overly sophisticated theoretical references, thus avoiding the risk that the student transfers them in an "adhesive" and forced way into his or her work with the patient. An important aspect of supervision, which has recently been highlighted by R. Romano Toscani (2017), is the quality of the interpersonal supervisor-trainee experience, which allows the transmission of the psychoanalytic technique. The supervisor and the supervisee build a bond of alliance between them, which overlaps the supervisee's alliance with the patient and which, in some respects, is isomorphic to the therapeutic relationship that develops between them as a parallel process; in this regard, G.O. Gabbard writes:

> The vulnerability of the supervisee in the relationship with the supervisor is in many respects comparable to the vulnerability of the patient in the therapeutic relationship … Instead, the supervisor has the task of creating an environment in which the therapist feels safe, willing to report frankly and directly what happens in the sessions with his patients.
>
> (2017)

As for the specific teaching function that develops in supervision, in general, we believe that supervision should help the supervisee to use the basic technical tools derived from classical psychoanalytic theory, adapting them to the context of psychoanalytic psychotherapy and stimulating, as a first and most important function, the student's intuitive and empathic abilities and attention to his/her own emotional responses, so as to foster understanding of transferential and counter-transferential movements. Equally appropriate is to encourage the student to pay attention to his/her patient's dreams, attempting an interpretation that integrates dream imagery, the patient's history and the course of therapy. The supervisee, when confronted with the psychotherapeutic task, must in turn learn to solicit in his/her patient attention to the imaginative-dream dimension, increasing his/her ability to recognize the Unconscious and become familiar with it, suggesting a symbolic/metaphorical reading of the facts narrated (Suman, 2008).

In supervision, the tools that characterize psychotherapy training and derive directly from our training are applied, for example, Infant Observation, which, as we have seen, calls for attention to the minutest details and non-verbal behaviour, and teaches the fundamental function of the observing and containing gaze. It is also important to encourage the correct use of clinical writing as a tool for the first reorganization in *après coup* of the thoughts on the case and the process that develops in the sessions, and the first elaboration that is then expanded upon in supervision. Working in supervision through writing makes it possible to reach blind areas of the relationship and to add new thoughts, thanks to the supervisor's *second glance* (Baranger, Baranger and Mom, 1993; Ferro, 1996). An example of this can be seen when the supervisee performs certain "slips" in writing resulting from unconscious transference movements, or even "suddenly" recalling certain pieces of the therapeutic dialogue only by re-reading the session report together with the supervisor. One aspect, finally, on which constant reflection and continuous monitoring by the supervisor are necessary, is the responsibility to respect the limits that require not entering the intimate sphere of the supervisee – an aspect that rather pertains to his or her analysis – but at the same time managing the emotional aspects that inevitably develop in supervision.

Supervision, in fact, is never only training, it is an emotional and affective experience that allows, in the *here and now* of supervision, the understanding and the constructive elaboration of the most intense affections and psychic pain that are present in the supervisee's relationship with the patient and that reverberate in supervision to be understood and reclaimed. We believe that this is the central aspect that makes supervision a cornerstone of the psychotherapist's training, along with his/her own analysis and theoretical study.

In our own training, as well as in the training we offer our students, both individual and group supervision are of great importance. Implemented in the AFPP from the outset, group supervision is conducted in small groups, in which each trainee presents a clinical case in consultation or psychotherapy; the material, presented in writing, after the reading becomes the subject of discussion by the participants, each of whom can ask for clarification, express their emotional responses, put forward personal thoughts about the material presented, and even refer to subjective experiences or take inspiration from similar cases in professional practice. A collaborative climate is created that tends to reconstruct new representations or narratives that, starting from the clinical case, activate the group's creative capacities. The group leader adopts the function of both moderating the participation of the interventions, attempting to formulate a synthesis of the contributions, integrating them into a general framework if possible, and of bringing his/her own contribution to the understanding of the case.

Notes

1 The lack of a reassuring social narrative of reality through meta-social and meta-psychological guarantors (a good family, clear social ethics, utopian solidarity, etc.) confronts individuals with a de-sublimated narrative (commercial war, primacy of money, competition for resources, etc.) that activates primary and undifferentiated states of the self (Biggio, 2022). Sociologists have been studying the loss of meta-social guarantors for a long time; for more on this topic, see the works of A. Touraine (1982) and E. Morin (1990).

2 At the National Conference on Psychoanalytic Psychotherapy "Contemporaneità e percorsi di sviluppo", organized by the SIPP in Rome in December 2017, Hansjorg Messner posed the question, present in the EFPP, of what is the most suitable setting to initiate a psychotherapeutic treatment, and what were the European criteria for the training of psychoanalytic psychotherapists.

3 Our group is trying to define the technical and methodological model that characterizes our psychotherapeutic approach. One of the most debated aspects is the use and interpretation of transference and counter-transference in psychoanalytic psychotherapy, with 1 or 2 weekly sessions ... What is your opinion on this? (Fano Cassese, 1987).

4 For a concise, but effective historical examination of this debate, see the article by A. Pazzagli (1992):

> Kleinian theory has never differentiated psychoanalytic psychotherapies from psychoanalysis, even though it holds at most to the purity of the setting and the rigour of the technique. The attempt to differentiate was more American, because in the USA there was a historical development of psychoanalysis in relation to psychiatry and the possibilities of psychotherapeutic intervention ... American culture ... has been a terrain in which psychoanalysis on the one hand has remained as the main activity, but on the other hand has generated a widespread use of therapies of various kinds that refer back to psychoanalysis.

5 Blatt and Shahar (2004). referring to research findings on the effect of therapist personality on long-term psychodynamic therapy, emphasize how "therapists' attachment styles can influence their professional relational mode and consequently the treatment process and effectiveness".

6 We cite, for example, a case in which the observer seemed to have functioned as a "container" of the mother's projective identifications, allowing her to internalize an experience of containment, which "lightened" her; this activated mental elaboration

processes of working through in the mother, which made it possible for her to recognize and communicate her difficulties, with consequent improvement in her relationship with the child.

7 Since the early 1980s, we have been discussing the multiple values and potentialities of Infant Observation with Livia Di Cagno, promoter of the diffusion and application of the method in Italy. Subsequently, from the 1990s to the present day, some of us have contributed to a vast international movement of in-depth study and comparison on the extension and use of this methodology in various fields. Numerous international and inter-continental meetings have been dedicated to the "extensions" of the IO method and its application in different contexts, including psychotherapy, in recent decades.

8 Isabella Lapi contributed to this paragraph.

References

Baranger, M., Baranger, W. and Mom, J.M. (1993). Processo e non processo nel lavoro analitico. *Ricerca Psicoanalitica*, VIII(1): 97–118.

Biggio, G. (2022). Trauma: Dissociazione sociale e individuale. *Contrappunto*, 62: 30–43.

Blatt, S.J. and Shahar, G. (2004). Psychoanalysis with Whom, for What, and How? Comparisons with Psychotherapy. *Journal of the American Psychoanalytic Association*, 52: 393–397.

Bolognini, S. (2018). Paper presented at the National Meeting of SIEFPP, Bologne (unpublished text).

Boston Change Process Study Group (2010). *Change in Psychotherapy: A Unifying Paradigm*. New York: W.W. Norton & Company.

Bromberg, P. (1998). *Standing in the Spaces: Essays on Clinical Process, Trauma, and Dissociation*. London: Routledge.

Fano Cassese, S. (1987). Dieci domande a Donald Meltzer. *Contrappunto*, 1: 43–46.

Ferrara Mori, G. (2001). Apprendere dall'osservazione: Excursus storico, riflessione e presupposti per un progetto di estensione della metodologia di Esther Bick. In L. Cresti, P. Farneti and C. Pratesi (eds), *Osservazione e trasformazione*. Rome: Borla.

Ferro, A. (1996). *Nella stanza d'analisi*. Milan: Raffaello Cortina.

Frisch, S., Hinshelwood, R.D. and Gauthier, J.M. (2001). *Psychoanalysis and Psychotherapy: The Controversies and the Future*. London: Karnac.

Gabbard, G.O. (2017). *Long-Term Psychodynamic Psychotherapy: A Basic Text*. 3rd edn. Washington, DC: American Psychiatric Publishing.

Gabbard, G.O. and Westen, D. (2003). Rethinking Therapeutic Action. *The International Journal of Psychoanalysis*, 84: 823–841.

Greenson, R. (1974). *The Technique and Practice of Psychoanalysis*. New York: International University Press Inc.

Grinberg, L. (1989). *La supervisione psicoanalitica. Teoria e pratica*. Milan: Raffaello Cortina.

Kernberg, O. (2003). Raccomandazioni per alcune innovazioni urgenti nella formazione psicoanalitica. *Gli Argonauti Rivista di Psicanalisi*, 97(3): 85–95.

McWilliams, N. (2019). *Il diniego: implicazioni sulle sue funzioni interne, relazionali, sociali e politiche*. Paper presented at National Meeting of the SIPP (unpublished text).

Morin, E. (1990). *Introduction à la pensée complexe*. Paris: ESF.

Mucci, C. (2020). *Corpi borderline. Regolazione affettiva e clinica dei disturbi di personalità*. Milan: Raffaello Cortina.

Nicolò, A.M. (2003). Utilità e limiti dell'interpretazione. In P. Fabozzi (ed.), *Forme dell'interpretare*. Milan: FrancoAngeli.

Nicolò, A.M. (2019). AI di là dell'interpretazione: Note sul cambiamento della tecnica in psicoanalisi. *Rivista di Psicoanalisi*, LXV(1): 815–834.

Pazzagli, A. (1992). Le psicoterapie psicoanalitiche: Borderline della psicoanalisi o entità autonoma? *Contrappunto*, 10: 9–19.

Ponsi, M. (2012). Portare alla coscienza l'inconscio? *Psiche: Rivista di cultura psicoanalitica*, Online, 1: 1–14.

Romano Toscani, R. (2017). *Conversazioni a due voci. Note sulla supervisione*. Milan: FrancoAngeli.

Suman, A. (1987). Editoriale. *Contrappunto*, 0: 1–6.

Suman, A. (2008). Note sulle supervisioni per psicoterapeuti, AFPP (unpublished text).

Suman, A. and Brignone, A. (2001). Psychoanalytic Psychotherapy and Psychoanalysis: A Choice in Step with the Times. In S. Frisch, R.D. Hinshelwood and J.N. Gauthier (eds), *Psychoanalysis and Psychotherapy: The Controversies and the Future*. London: Karnac.

Touraine, A. (1982). *La produzione della società*. Bologne: Il Mulino.

Turillazzi Manfredi, S. (1979). *La linea d'ombra delle psicoterapie*. Florence: Del Riccio.

Wallerstein, R. (2001). Foreword. In S. Frisch, R.D. Hinshelwood and J.N. Gauthier (eds), *Psychoanalysis and Psychotherapy: The Controversies and the Future*. London: Karnac.

Chapter 2

Non-interpretive therapeutic factors

Containing functions in the therapeutic relationship

Luigia Cresti

In Chapter 1, we offered a brief overview of the rapid changes that have taken place in the social, cultural and existential context that characterises today's reality and of their influence on the type of psychological suffering that results also at an individual level.[1] The loss of meta-social guarantors has been followed by the loss of meta-psychic guarantors, determining new forms of malaise that we are called upon to deal with. What is required, therefore, is a shift in perspective in considering the problems and personological characteristics of the patients who currently come to us, using a different viewpoint than the one adopted in the diagnostic classifications we usually refer to.

In this context, it is a common observation that many of the people who come to us for psychotherapy often present conditions of indistinct malaise, identity indefiniteness, and disturbance of the sense of self, rather than circumscribed conflictual nuclei of a neurotic type, or a serious psychotic dysfunction. Even the phenomenon, already mentioned, of gender "fluidity", which frequently comes to our attention, especially in our work with adolescents, suggests that the original internal references of these people are marked by indefiniteness and lability, and that there is an uncertain, undefined structuring of the self as its basis. In these patients, the relationship with their emotional world often seems precluded or poorly articulated, as if they had not learnt the language of affection and their discomfort is mainly translated into bodily states or enactments. We could say, in other words, that at the basis of these multiple problems there is a defect or inadequate constitution of the internal container (understood as the structure that defines the Self).

The fact is that with many of these patients, it is not indicated to resort *tout court* to the interpretation of transference and specific conflictual contents, as in the classical psychoanalytic model. On the contrary, a work (preliminary, but not only) of construction/strengthening/stabilisation of the internal container is required, but this is only possible starting from the constitution of the external/therapeutic container, which can then gradually be internalised. With this, our attention shifts to the appropriate therapeutic interventions to deal with these different psychopathological configurations and focuses on the overriding importance of the *containing function of the therapeutic relationship*, in its

DOI: 10.4324/9781032673721-3

multiple declinations. It is precisely on the non-interpretive therapeutic factors that our interest as psychotherapists has focused. As an introduction to the development of this theme, I will introduce a brief historical-theoretical digression on the notion of *containment*.

The therapeutic container

It is necessary to define more precisely what is meant by containment, outlining its conceptual references and the functions it performs in the clinic. In fact, the term "containment" is so often used in the jargon of theory and clinical practice that it appears ubiquitous, with the risk of sometimes becoming approximate and generic, a sort of passe-partout useful to describe multiple processes: it offers an explanatory model of the child's psycho-affective development, of therapeutic intervention, of the functions that can be carried out by empathic observation and the supportive/integrative function carried out by the family, the group, the institution, and so on. It may therefore be useful to rethink the multiple meanings that this notion implies, by concisely reviewing the main conceptual formulations in this regard and their repercussions in clinical practice.

The concept of container developed first of all in the English area of thought, where it assumed a central meaning for all addresses of psychoanalytical psychotherapy, both within and outside the Kleinian group. The idea of container derives from the original Kleinian description (Klein, 1952) of projective identification (whereby one person "contains" a part of another); from this then derived a theory of development based on the emotional contact of the baby with the mother and, by extension, a theory of psychoanalytic contact. It is well known that we are indebted to W. Bion (1962) for the mature formulation of this model: he understood that the early infantile emotional states are experienced concretely and therefore cannot be used for mental growth. In order for them to be transformed into something that can be thought, imagined, remembered (i.e., to become alpha elements), there must be identification with a container-object, capable of receiving the chaos and confusion that the child experiences concretely and of responding to it creatively, making him feel that the intolerable can be tolerated: this is the fundamental function of rêverie. Containment therefore refers to the mother's capacity to receive the child's projective identifications and to return them after having modified them and made them fit for integration; this allows the transformation of a distressing experience to which a meaning can be given and allows the passage from beta elements to alpha elements, that is to say, to leave the level of the sensorial, somatic state to access mentalisation. "Containing" means that the mother can modify the distressing experience and return it to the infant in the form of order and harmony, from which the catastrophic anxiety has been removed (the alpha function). Bion insists that rêverie responses must be offered repeatedly and over a long period of time in order for them to be truly introjected by the infant. This process whereby the mother's rêverie enables her to give a response to the infant's projections functions similarly in the analytic situation; the therapist's rêverie also enables the mentalisation of the experience and provides the psychic tools to keep the scattered parts of the personality together. The container thus has a dynamic and organising role, which is not limited to a passive function, but operates an effective transformation of the psychic elements. H. Segal (1957 [1984]) took up this idea, making it the basis of the technique of treatment with severely distressed patients. She argued that a patient can construct an ego through the introjection of an object capable of containing and understanding experiences.

If in the Bionian meaning of *containment* the idea of understanding and transforming the child's (or patient's) suffering into a mental one prevails, the implications of Winnicott's *holding* are different. According to D.W. Winnicott (1961), in fact, holding refers to bodily acts full of psychological values, with which the mother-environment holds and supports the child, thus allowing it to acquire a unitary state, so that the psyche can settle in the soma. The notion of containing implicit in holding is given by the fact that the mother, with her empathy-laden physical care, gives the baby a feeling of cohesion and favours the development of a sense of continuity of being. The structuring value of the holding, however, refers not only to the initial stages of the individual's psycho-affective development: the ego's support continues to be a necessity for the growing child, for the adolescent and also for the adult, whenever there is a tension that threatens to confuse and disintegrate him. For Winnicott, the holding concept is also very useful in describing social work in the sense that disintegrating forces in individuals, but also in families and individual social groups, can be counteracted by offering a *holding environment* to children, adolescents with anti-social tendencies, psychiatric patients, etc.

In therapy, holding means offering the patient a relational continuity with a person who is empathically interested in understanding. In *Psychoanalytic Explorations*, Winnicott states that "for some patients the fact of structuring and maintaining the setting is more important than the interpretative work" (1964 [1985]), that is, the setting is seen as a real element for the formation and support of the self.

We know how E. Bick (1964) developed the Bionian idea of containment by describing the psychic function of the skin in the context of mental development. For psychic growth it is necessary to experience an object that contains, the baby must feel sufficiently contained within the skin, understood in the physical and psychic sense at the same time, which constitutes a sort of protective membrane that will then be gradually internalised. From the repeated internalisation of the containing object an internal psychic space can be constituted within which objects can be received and introjected, thus initiating a three-dimensional functioning: the therapy room protects the patient from sensations that are too vivid; the regularity of the schedule and the fairly long duration of the session mitigate the discontinuity produced by the variations in psychic and organic rhythms.

The notion of "psychic skin" was then taken up and expanded by D. Anzieu (1974), who, starting from the theoretical data of various orders of studies as well as from the psychosomatic investigation of dermatological disorders, elaborated the notion of *ego-skin*, which was later enriched in that of *enveloppe*. [2] Anzieu's aim is to investigate the precocious modalities of the transformation of primitive bodily experiences, believing that in psychoanalytic technique one must pay different attention to the phenomena that can be traced back to the *skin enveloppe*: that is, the analyst, like a mother, must learn to grasp and accept what the patient essentially expresses with bodily experiences, in order to be able to then transform them, returning them to the patient with their meaning; this implies a particular exercise of the therapist's observational skills. Anzieu's thinking (Anzieu et al., 1987) is based on the fact that, in his experience, many of the patients who require treatment are borderline patients or narcissistic personalities, and this requires technical adjustments and conceptual innovations that allow a better clinical understanding. These patients are suffering from:

> a lack of limits, an uncertainty of boundaries between the corporeal and the psychic ... of abrupt fluctuations of these boundaries accompanied by lapses into depression ... of a confusion between pleasant and painful experiences ... All this makes the faults of the psychic *enveloppe* evident: a widespread feeling of malaise, a sense of not living one's own life, of being a spectator of something that is not one's own existence ... It is necessary, therefore, to develop conceptual tools that allow one to reconstruct limits and re-establish frontiers such that the territories of belonging that can be inhabited within the self can be identified.
>
> (Anzieu et al., 1987)

In terms of treatment, this means that becoming aware of the container constitutes an indispensable stage in understanding the ego faults; only in this way can one arrive at the reconstruction of the traumatisms that occurred in the early relationship and that produced the distortions of the psychic *enveloppe*. Before interpreting the drive conflict, the therapist must therefore work on the alterations of the psychic containers.

The concept of *"enveloppe"*, introduced by Anzieu in 1974, was taken up and deepened in French psychoanalysis, in the wake of the observation that the new clinical contexts (psychoanalytic treatment of children, of "borderline states", of the family and of groups) directed attention to the structures that delimit and contain, that is, to the "containers" as well as to the "contents" (fantasies, affects, internal objects), as was traditionally the case in classical psychoanalysis. The basic hypothesis of this different therapeutic approach is that in the session the patient projects his own psychic *enveloppe*, through modes of communication that are for the most part primitive. The term "*enveloppe*" implies both aspects of the patient's mental functioning and of the "analytic framework" (Bleger, 1967), that is, it indicates both a structural aspect of the individual's psyche and the object or place into which the subject's drives and fantasies are conveyed through projective identification.

Remaining in the French area of thought, an important contribution was made by D. Houzel, who, in his in-depth reflection on the containing functions in therapy, states:

> In situations of dispersion, turbulence, chaos … a process of organising the emotional drives must first be initiated before one can think about the elaboration of emotional conflicts in the transference; this process is made possible by the constitution of an enveloppe, which is provided by the containing aspects of the therapeutic framework.

> (1987)

Although they are based on different visions of the mental and relational processes involved in psychoanalytic therapy, these conceptual formulations are, however, united by the emphasis on the importance of the functions of acceptance, resilience, coherence and reliability that many patients prioritise.

With regard then to the non-interpretive therapeutic tools that appear most appropriate in the situations mentioned above, it is basically a matter of offering the patient:

- stability, regularity, continuity of the relationship with the therapist (which recalls the Winnicottian idea of the setting as a holding environment);
- attentive, empathic, interested listening to the anxieties, thoughts, feelings verbalised by the patient;
- observation and attribution of meaning to all of the patient's manifestations (including non-verbal ones), so as to broaden the area of "meanings" and make the sphere of emotions more accessible.

An example of an external container

We present a clinical flash, from a brief psychotherapy of a little girl who has undergone a serious trauma. This case shows the containing function given by the setting, the gaze and the listening; this function seems to somehow extend to the mother who waits outside the room. The process of setting construction and its predictability are the track on which the psychotherapy with little Fiona runs. Her need to be listened to, welcomed, but above all "seen", meant that the encounters quickly became effective. One is reminded of the constantly repeated mode of speech of children who, with each new achievement and acquisition of skills, need to repeat "… mummy, look … teacher, look …". The things that happen and the discoveries made are not really such if they are not seen and named, that is, if they are not given a meaning by someone entrusted with the task of attesting and naming them, thus making them exist.

Fiona: "I was shouting, but they couldn't see me!"

Fiona[3] (4½ years old) was attacked and severely bitten in the face by a dog; the child is a little blond cyclone dragging the adult towards her world and fantasies, through play and relationship/communication. She takes total possession of the room and the toys; with frequency and naturalness, she glides quickly to the desk and, without forcing, quietly and softly, sits on the therapist's legs and looks carefully at the objects and the room from this perspective, as if she wanted to make the therapist's gaze her own. She does not intrude forcefully, nor does she touch the objects aggressively, rather she touches them as if they were her own. She refuses to talk about the traumatic event: "The fears? I no longer have them, they have passed, but I always have new ones ...". In the first session, she drew a sky and underneath a meadow, leaving a large part of the sheet blank in the middle and commenting that she could not find enough space to draw her father: "... I wanted to draw my family, but it doesn't fit". The next time, when the therapist invites her again to talk about her fears, she replies firmly: "Later... when you draw." From session to session to the first almost empty drawing with lots of white space, Fiona adds characters and details, evidence of the progressive formation of a container that can accommodate her thoughts and emotions. At this point, the therapist feels that Fiona can finally talk about her fears and the thoughts that come into her head and tells her that when one is afraid, one stands still but has many thoughts. Then Fiona re-enacts the scene of herself on the ground and the dog that bites her in the face, saying: "... I was screaming for help but they couldn't see me, then a teacher saw me. But now I am beautiful again! Look!" The gaze of the Other – of the teacher who finally sees, of the therapist who observes – saves by bringing help. Afterwards, Fiona declares that she will draw a picture, that it will be for the therapist, and that she will leave it with her (the previous ones she demanded to take them away), saying that she will draw many more things on it in the future. The mother who waits outside and always arrives in a hurry tells me that she doesn't know what's going on "there in the room, but it's good for me too because while I'm waiting I relax and even take a nap". In the following meetings, Fiona's drawings became increasingly rich in detail and an explosion of bright colours, ending with a very colourful drawing in which "mummy is doing a dance show". After about six months, at the closing meeting agreed upon and announced to both her and her parents, Fiona, when asked how she is doing, replies: "You have to face your fears and then I came to you!" She takes the note with the therapist's telephone number, "... what if Mummy loses it?", and says goodbye.

The therapist's gaze and the visual *enveloppe*

The aspect of participant observation – as already mentioned in Chapter 1 – occupies a peculiar place and is charged with a particularly significant value in psychoanalytic psychotherapy, where most interventions are carried out precisely in the face-to-face modality. We intend, of course, the term "observation" not in the sense of a simple perceptive act, with cognitive-exploratory aims, but in the sense of an empathic, receptive function, which is based on identification with the patient's needs, also through attention to one's own counter-transference: that observational modality, in short, which we have learnt through the prolonged exercise of Infant Observation, according to E. Bick.

In my experience, I have found over the years that the relationship of participant observation that is established between the observer and the mother-baby couple, while not having therapeutic aims (Brutti and Brutti, 1996) and does not envisage the use of interventions of an interpretative type, can sometimes perform an implicit transformative function with respect to the mother, the child and their mutual relationship, in that processes are activated that may constitute the premises for an improvement of their relationship; In this regard, I will mention a case (which I supervised in the Infant Observation training of the AFPP) in which the observer seemed to have functioned as a depository of the mother's projective identifications, allowing her to internalise an experience of containment, which relieved her. This activated mental elaboration processes in the mother that made it possible for her to recognise and communicate her own difficulties, with a consequent improvement in her relationship with the child.

Various authors have explored the issue of the transformative potential of observation: M. Pérez-Sanchez (1982) spoke of the observer's gaze as an "inward-looking gaze" that solicits in parents an interest in the child's internal world; G. Ferrara Mori (2001) highlighted how contact with the observer's non-verbal but mental functions, with her sustained attention and her gaze, allows the child and his family to make an initial transformation of their emotional experiences and helps to contain painful experiences instead of evacuating them. We too have addressed these issues in various writings (Cresti and Lapi, 1996; Cresti, 1997).

In adopting this perspective, I verified that even in our clinical experience as psychotherapists, the therapeutic process often seems to be initiated by those same relational factors that can lend support and "cure" value to observation and that have to do primarily with the containing functions of eye contact.

But what, more precisely, are the containing aspects of the therapeutic framework related to observation?

• The therapist may perform an implicit task of being a "receptacle" of the patient's projective identifications, analogous to what sometimes happens in the relationship between the observer and the mother (I mentioned above, for example, some problematic observational situations in which there seems to have been an easing of the mother's malaise, through the "evacuation" of parts of the suffering self into an external object, the participant observer).[4] This function of the therapist/observer corresponds to what Meltzer (1967) described as the "toilet-breast".

• The therapist's observational attitude, thanks to the "receptive" values of his or her attentive and sensitive gaze, can facilitate the initiation of transformative processes in the direction of a better integration, delimitation, and coherence of the sense of self.

Such integrative/supportive implications of the visual relationship have been variously theorised by several authors. I will limit myself here to citing M. Harris, according to whom, observation "helps the patient to bind his words and actions together in a more meaningful way ... to organise his anxieties, to contain and diminish disintegrative effects" (1987); G. Haag, who connotes the gaze (of the observer or of the therapist, in the treatment of children) as "a force that magnetises, attracts, collects ... In intense moments of interrelation, it plays a unifying role, integrating the other sensory and sensual modalities" (1988). In short, the patient benefits from what French authors (D. Anzieu, D. Houzel, G. Haag) call *enveloppe visuel*, a "wrapping" that contains, supports and delimits.

I will now try to elaborate on the implications of the eye contact between therapist and patient: Analysing the meaning that the relationship with the face and especially the gaze of the therapist, who offers himself to the patient in the face-to-face setting, can assume, we can imagine that the therapist's attentive and participating gaze (together with facial expressions), functioning as an organ and spokesperson of the mind, performs first of all a receptive task (in that it welcomes, letting them pass in, a whole series of extra-verbal signs to which a meaning can be attributed), offering precisely a "visually containing framework". But, in addition to this, one can imagine that it also conveys a sort of "restitution" of the therapist's understanding and participation. As Correale states (Correale et al., 1994), in order to facilitate the process of reintegration of projections, the therapist must function as a container and mirror. In my opinion, this statement condenses a more Bionian vertex (the mimic expression and the therapist's face transmit his ability to tolerate emotions, offering a "transformative restitution" of the anxieties transmitted by the patient); at the same time one can think, in a Winnicottian perspective, of a function of mirroring of affects, which makes it possible for the patient to feel recognised and supported in deep aspects of the Self.[5]

We further explore the transformative functions of the gaze (both in observation of the mother-child pair and in therapy), through the teaching of T.H. Ogden:

> The child in his mother's eyes does not simply see himself mirrored but sees himself transformed in his mother's eyes, sees his mother's interpretation of

him … not his mirror image (his double). Rather, what he sees is her impression of him, the mark he has made on another person, an impression with which the mother, in turn, has built something.

(2016)

It is thus the experience of a connection with another other than oneself, which opens, albeit in a non-verbal form, to the development of the symbolic functions of the mind and to self-awareness. Similarly, through his "mental" gaze, the therapist transmits to the patient meanings that interpret the internal world and the emotional exchange that occurs in the session, promoting in him a possible therapeutic change. The following clinical cases briefly illustrate some of the therapeutic components related to the face-to-face treatment, discussed so far.

In the case that follows, that of Paolo, the therapist's non-verbal behavioural signals activate in the boy the ability to see emotions, showing how the patient not only can feel recognised in the emotions manifested by the Other, but also learn that certain emotions exist, and then discover them, little by little, within himself.

Paolo: tears in my eyes

Paolo[6] is a 12-year-old boy who has developed a serious behavioural disorder, accompanied by addiction to video games, which manifests itself in aggressive acting out towards his parents, even to the point of hitting them at times not directly related to video game excitement or in response to imposed restrictions or arguments with them. The concern is great for both parents and therapist because several months after the start of therapy, not only is there no improvement, but the situation even appears to be worsening. The one-week sessions are completely occupied by filling sheets and sheets of scribbles in red felt-tip pen where Paolo describes himself killing his mother, burning her, cutting her to pieces, throwing her out of the window, shooting her, and ending with squiggles that cover everything, cancelling out any white space, sometimes to the point of soaking the paper in ink and violently piercing it. The counter-transference is one of great anxiety and of no use is the verbalisation of feelings that the boy does not seem to listen to, or that he actively rejects by intensifying the anger, the darts with the felt-tip pen and the provocative affirmations of homicidal intentions. One day, Paolo arrives at the session after yet another physical confrontation with his mother: she bursts into the room, saying that she can't take it any longer and that she will send Paolo away from home, looking for a community for him; Paolo looks shattered, very pale and weak as if he were about to fall asleep or faint. The therapist finds herself invaded and attacked by the violence emanating from them and feels within herself a deep discouragement, never before felt so intensely. The session passes wearily, with Paulo alternating between moments of anger exploded by punching and tearing papers and moments in which he slumps inertly in his chair; at no time during the session does the boy agree to talk about what happened, and he shushes the therapist if she tries to verbalise anything. On the way home after the session, however, Paulo suddenly says to his mother, in a tone not of defiance but of curiosity, "You know, doctor Lapi was just about to cry." The mother is struck by this statement and, feeling that it is somehow important, immediately phones the therapist to tell her.

We can think that the therapist's reaction, spontaneous and sincere, which was channelled directly to the boy through the body, was a kind of teaching that intrigued him: the existence of strong emotions such as pain and despair that annihilate, emotions that he could not find within himself but whose existence he could learn and recognise through the tears in the therapist's eyes. These were a message that touched him in a more direct, stronger, more evident way than words, which triggered a progressive internal transformation.

In the following session, a character appears for the first time in one of his drawings, his grandmother's cat, whom Paulo says he loves, and whom he represents in the act of eating. The therapist then asks who does the cooking in his house, and in the conversation that follows, the figure of his mother appears who makes, particularly "very good cakes", while his father does the shopping. At last an opening has opened up where different emotions other than rage and murderous fury can pass, and good aspects of internal objects can be recovered.

Alina: the empty mirror

The case of Alina,[7] a 16-year-old girl who came in for treatment for an eating disorder (self-induced vomiting and refusal of food), shows how, from the very beginning of the therapeutic relationship, the young patient's need to make use of the containing functions offered by the therapist's empathic gaze was central. Participatory observation, in its countertransferential values, led on my part to an attribution of meaning to the patient's multiple messages, including bodily and non-verbal ones, favouring a better integration of her psychic *enveloppe*.

In Alina's story, an early defect of family containment was evident, in the sense of a deficiency and inconsistency of the parental functions of attention and empathic care. The mother, a dull woman, fragile and prone to depression, had had many difficulties with the child since her pregnancy and had taken little care of her; the marriage had lasted only a short time and Alina had lived alternately with her mother or father, witnessing confused erotic-sentimental relationships of both parents with other partners. In the initial meeting I had with Alina and her mother, I was unpleasantly struck by the fact that the latter was little able to focus on the milestones and significant aspects of her daughter's growth and rather tended to talk a lot about her own difficult childhood as an orphan. Alina's condition, as a neglected child and an adolescent unseen and left to her own devices, as well as her own fragile and delicate physical appearance, immediately induced in me a particularly intense countertransference, full of sorrow and solicitude at the same time. In the third therapy session, the girl described to me her feelings about food, saying that she could enjoy the taste of it in her mouth, but could not tolerate the food being inside, so she felt an urgent need to throw it out. I then proposed that she draw me a picture telling me how she felt at those times and she drew, to my surprise, a picture of herself in front of a large empty mirror: a mirror described by her as a "monster" that did not reflect her image, perceived as hostile and distancing, in front of which she represented herself with unclear contours. With this drawing and the verbalisation that accompanied it, Alina seemed to tell me of her suffering for not having been able to benefit from the experience of empathic mirroring carried out by the maternal gaze (Winnicott, 1967 [1974]) and, at the same time, to address an implicit request, in the transference, that I function for her as a "mirroring gaze" that looks, welcomes, thinks, giving her back a more defined image of herself, invested with affective meaning and libidinal value. I therefore believed I sensed that the containment offered by a participating and interested gaze constituted a necessary condition for her so that the therapeutic nourishment could also be received within, rather than rejected.

The importance, for this girl, of feeling seen, looked at, and focused on, often returned in the sessions as a leitmotif: at times, she communicated to me her sorrow at having hardly ever been photographed by her parents, not even in childhood; or she had me read her poems, dedicated to her mother, on the suffering that her "cold eyes ... the glassy, soulless gaze" caused her. I was very impressed by the verbal content brought to the sessions by this sensitive girl, but at the same time I realised that a particular attention was mobilised in me on certain aspects, especially the type of glances and smiles with which she gradually presented herself at the sessions. Sometimes it was precisely these messages (especially the quality of Alina's glances at me) that oriented my countertransference and guided my interventions; for her part, the girl also seems to have experienced my interest in looking at her with attention and empathy, as an experience of reciprocity and attribution of meaning, which would perhaps have been less intense in the absence of the face-to-face experience. I believe that the offer of this visual containment helped to initiate a process of recognition and organisation of her emotions, which then developed further in the therapeutic relationship.

Giulia: the gazes that meet

The case of Giulia[8] shows the mirroring of the gaze in the therapeutic relationship and its internalised containing function. Giulia was brought to me at the age of 8 by her adoptive parents because of a series of behavioural difficulties which, in therapy, soon became the evident and disconcerting signs of an incipient perverse personality organisation: sadism, pornography, and falsification of the truth were rampant in the sessions, which appeared to be the consequence of early experiences of affective deprivation and traumatism (the original family context was chaotic, murky and abusive). In the succession of sessions, I felt for a long time the difficulty of making intimate contact with this child, who protected herself from the anguish of trauma with a shell of apparent cynicism and harshness. In the second year of therapy, however, there was an unexpected positive change in the emotional climate, through a change in the quality of the messages conveyed by the looks. In other words, a two-way relational process began whereby the little girl was able to open up to the internal world and to affective implication thanks to the possibility, offered to her, of grasping authentic emotional meanings in the therapist's gaze. It could be said that the eyes functioned as a vehicle for a complex game of projective identifications on the part of the little girl and countertransferential responses on the part of the therapist. During a session, Giulia told the sad story of a 4-year-old child who lost his parents and was left alone; this account made me feel emotional (she had in fact been given up for adoption at the age of 4!). I emphasise the painfulness of the story that perhaps reminds her of something she had also experienced. The little girl, looking at me with amazement in her eyes, which were probably a bit tearful because of compassion, asks me why I feel like crying and she insistently inquires what I feel and why. She then confesses her need to understand more about her story; she would really like me, in agreement with her adoptive mother, to fill in the gaps in her story. She then comments, as if speaking to herself, that friendship is a very important thing in life... She then fills a rubber balloon with lukewarm water and plays at "feeding" from it; faced with my reference to the possibility of a good breastfeeding experience, she replies: "That's the tit, warm to the point!" At the end of the hour she leaves, kissing me.

The fact that the little girl perceived the countertransferential response, expressed by the quality of my gaze, full of compassion and tenderness, seems to have allowed her the experience of feeling recognised and welcomed in the denied aspects of herself, in a truer emotional dimension and of finding within herself a new space of relationship and resonance. In a later session, the girl drew "The gazes that meet" (Figure 2.1) and wrote me a "poem" in which she tried to explain her confused and conflicting feelings, related to the fear of abandonment, and her defensive need to resort to arousal and pornographic thoughts.

These cases help us to understand how the gaze that welcomes, understands and participates can facilitate making contact with deep feelings and make possible – as Meltzer (1967) puts it – the "opening to the luminosity of the internal space". This can activate a process that is not only containing, but also transformative, of progress in mentalisation, i.e., becoming a valuable working tool for the therapist who can use it to explore the patient's deep

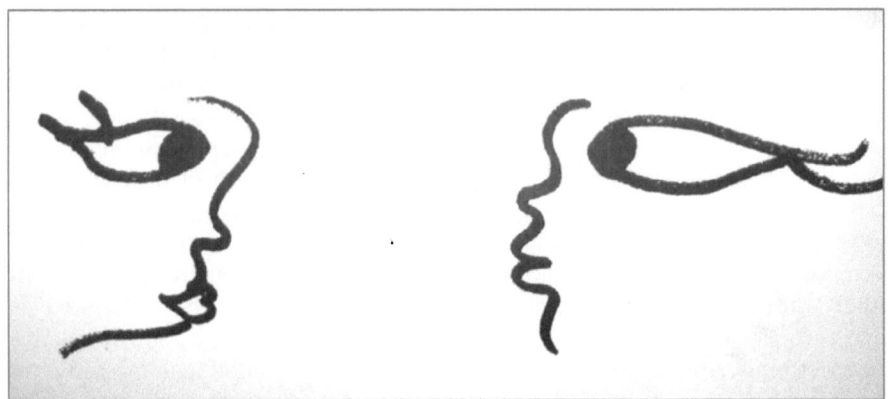

Figure 2.1 The gazes that meet

emotional experience and to promote change, as sometimes happens in the Infant Observation experience.

The sound *enveloppe*: sound messages and the musical dimension of transference

What has been said about the function of a containing and delimiting *enveloppe* implied in the gaze also relates to the sound aspects of the therapeutic relationship. On the therapist's side it is important to listen "musically" to the sound messages, verbal and non-verbal, sent by the patient, as this can help the therapist grasp and re-signify deep and original aspects; but also on the patient's side, the relationship with the therapist's voice as a carrier of emotions can be important, as it allows an experience of containment through the constitution of a sound *enveloppe*.

Marta: an envelopping *voice*

Marta,[9] 12 years old, at the beginning of a session, after about a year and a half of therapy, told me that after the previous session she had been particularly well, that she had returned home relieved and satisfied, but that she absolutely could not relate to anything I had said to her, but rather to the tone of my voice that had enveloped and cradled her, leaving her with a deep sense of well-being. I thought that the patient was able to enjoy the "cuddling" sound of my voice for the first time, without this activating persecutory experiences in her. She was able in therapy to experience a previously unknown affective dimension.

Even in adult therapy, M. Mancia (1998) has greatly emphasised the importance of the "musical dimension" of transference; before that, Meltzer (1967) illustrated the value of "musicality" in transference. The sound messages sent by the therapist can in part protect the patient from primitive anxieties of loss of limits and control, allowing contact with primitive states of the mind, otherwise hardly contactable. D. Anzieu and D. Houzel (1987), on the subject of the original roots of the ego, proposed the idea of considering "sound space" as the first psychic space. This space seems to be constructed in therapy before words, providing a warm, enveloping container that allows the transference relationship to begin.

Rosa: a warming voice

Rosa,[10] unexpectedly, at the end of a session, tells the therapist: "You know, I don't listen to the words you tell me. It's not that I don't understand them: it's that they don't mean anything. But I hear the tone in which you speak to me and that gets to me. It's like I'm all frozen up inside, but the way you speak to me I feel it melts something in me." Through the sound and tone of the therapist's voice, Rosa can thus find a "consonance", a shared basis for communication and a more authentic and trusting relationship.

In the psychotherapy of severely ill patients, a strong need is particularly evident for a sound container to be created in the sessions to calm their anguish of emptiness; especially in the first phase of psychotherapy, they become distressed if silences are produced that are long and forlorn for them. They need to hear the sound of words or even, simply, that the therapist "produces sounds", which may not necessarily be vocal. "But even in cases where the personality deterioration is minor, the importance of the therapist's voice is evident, and it becomes an important field of projections and introjections" (Sabsay Foks, 1998).

Sonia: a cradling voice

Sonia[11] is a young adult diagnosed with schizophrenia. Although she regularly comes to the sessions, she appears very frightened of the relationship and closed in her delusional world. For a long, long time, the sessions are filled with her incessant psychotic confabulations, without pauses, which the therapist can only hear and, at most, punctuate with words like "hum", "yes", "ah". At a certain point, brief moments of silence begin to appear in the sessions, which the therapist can start to speak to her; these spaces become gradually longer and more frequent, during which Sonia finally seems to listen. The therapist's words at this point are accepted and appreciated for their sound that Sonia shows she perceives regressing to a precocious infantile state that makes her say: "How pleasant it is to be with Mummy listening to songs ... doing something together."

The therapeutic container, at first perceived by Sonia only in its more concrete physical aspects (the room, the start and end time of the session), is enriched with the therapist's words, first heard for their musicality, then, as if transported by sound, gradually listened to in their content as well.

The musicality of the voice in online psychotherapeutic consultations
Isabella Lapi

> Music teaches us the most important thing there is:
>   listening.
>
> Ezio Bosso

In the sound *enveloppe*, the voice acquires a central function not only through the words that communicate content but also through its musical components that reach the emotional world directly, with particular intensity when other sensory channels are absent. The experience of online psychotherapeutic consultations, carried out during the pandemic,[12] most often by telephone, confirmed the function of the musicality of the voice in creating the possibility of listening and being listened to, soothing distress, transmitting support. Despite having the choice of whether to make the consultations by video call or phone call only, many people preferred to use the telephone. If the choice for some, especially if they were elderly, was due to their being less familiar with other communication devices ("no, no, doctor, let's leave these means to the young"), for others, it stemmed from mistrust of talking to a stranger. Only in a few cases did this diffidence take on tones of reticence concealing fears of a persecutory type (expressed, for example, in wanting to give only one's first name or to be vague in specifying one's address), while in the majority, it was given by understandable caution in having to talk about intimate experiences with a stranger, and also by perceiving the video as somewhat invasive of private space. In reality, caution disappeared almost immediately, often during the very first interview, because the voice succeeded in creating an immediate bond: "thank you, the sound of your voice reassured me", "what a beautiful voice", "I am glad to hear from you again soon"; the voice soon acquired a calming function: "your voice makes me feel good", and it lessened feelings of loneliness: "When I feel lonely I think of your voice", "I have been waiting since the morning to hear your voice". The words "phone call", "conversation", "interview" were almost never used, in the absence of visual communication and the need to bridge the distance,[13] the voice was the element perceived as central, almost unique in importance, especially in moments of greatest distress.

The most frequent way of communicating between people is through the voice, a vehicle of emotions, rich on a non-verbal level with infinite nuances and qualities: The voice in itself can be an affect, a fantasy ... the voice, as sound, brings us closer to the primary process than structured language, which instead depends on the secondary process"(Mancia, 1998).[14]

The voice itself has the power to overcome barriers and eliminate distances:

> Visual perception, like auditory, is distal. However, in terms of distance, the auditory does not encompass the distance that the visual can encompass. Voice can be used, then, to eliminate the distance between speaker and receptor. On the one hand, both the voice emitting into the other (projection) and the reciprocal, can represent an object in itself.
>
> (Sabsay Foks, 1998)

The voice as a "sound object" laden with affectivity is created in the pre-verbal communication of the primary relationship between mother and child, who is sensitive to the musicality of the mother's voice; similarly, in therapy, there is a pre-verbal level in the communication between therapist and patient, who shows great sensitivity to the therapist's voice; Mauro Mancia writes on this subject:

> I have defined this as the musical dimension of the transference, which forces the analyst to develop a particular form of rêverie, that is, what can be called an acoustic rêverie. The analyst is no longer merely the one who must decode a narrative, transforming it into its metaphorical equivalent, but is also the one who must be able to use the infraverbal and musical aspect of communication.
>
> (Mancia, 2004)[15]

The voice as a sound object in early relationships and in the psychotherapeutic relationship evocatively takes us even further back, to the early experience of the uterine container, which envelops, keeps warm and protects, where the lights and noises of the world arrive blurred and muffled, made tolerable by the protection of the uterine walls, and where the sounds of the mother's heartbeat, the inside of her body and her voice prevail. On these sensory experiences, the first sketches of internal objects are built.[16]

We may therefore think that in telephone consultations the patients experienced a good sound *enveloppe* offered by the therapist's voice that sends them back to reassuring early experiences. The sound-induced regression opened up intimacy where confidences could be expressed that were rich in intense emotion and sometimes violent in their psychic pain. The therapist was also very emotionally involved, sometimes induced to close his/her eyes not so much to concentrate as to live the same experience of sound contact and regression as the other. In the short- and long-distance consultations required by supporting interventions during the pandemic, the therapist was forced to do without the usual working tools, such as extended time and the possibility of interpreting, and to make much more use of herself and her own observation and listening skills, but in the telephone consultations, she was faced with the new situation of doing without even her gaze and those visual data that are so useful to build up an image of the patient and his problems. The therapist, perhaps in order to make up for this deprivation, found herself fantasising about the person on the other end of the telephone, paying much more attention than usual to modulating the intonation of the voice and the rhythm of the speech, listening with participation to the Other's silences while measuring out her own. A. Ferruta, in an intervention on silence in analysis, with the eloquent title "Silence is someone who listens", suggests thinking of silence as a way of access to:

> something that is not immediately perceptible ... something that is born while listening to one who is capable of silencing his own narcissism to meet the other, to listen to the unknown voice, never heard ... The analysis opens up to listening to those creative notes that spring from an encounter, in the disappearance of explanations and prescriptions, to make way for sound, dance, the evocative word of poetry. An analyst who listens to the crunching of snow and leaves under the feet of a subject who moves in the world, who is not immobilised in a diagnosis or in a transference relationship that coercively repeats. It requires listening and creative passion.
>
> (2012)

In the consultations, silences, in the absence of sensory and visual perceptions, were felt as highly significant, substantial, important to understand, to respect, to give rhythm to, perhaps even more difficult to tolerate, since they evoked deprivation and loss. Within a relationship built with only the sound of the voice, with breathing, at times with sobbing, it was as if the silences acquired a musical value of their own, like pauses within a score, in which the music is suspended, allowing the listener to reflect, to rethink what he or she has heard, and then to continue, to resume the suspended theme and listen to it again, or to go on to new sonorities, silences not empty of sounds, but pause-silences full of thoughts and listening, silence-spaces to express and understand. Silences that alone allow us to listen to the faintest sounds such as the crunching of snow or the sound of leaves!

The suffering of people who telephoned was often described as a sense of loneliness and emptiness, loss and bereavement, and "feeling in a dark tunnel in which you can't see the light" was the metaphor used by many; yet, the telephone call immediately seemed to brighten the darkness because the sound of the voice testified to the active presence of someone.[17]

Some patients from the regressive darkness filled only by the sound of the voice, set off on a path towards the light, regaining possession of renewed and more confident ego capacities: at the end of the consultation, it was not uncommon, in fact, to find the desire and the possibility of a more complete relational contact. Adding visual contact to sound contact had for some the purpose of fixing the memory in the mind, for instance, through photos: "may

I send you the photo of me with my grandchildren?", "I saw your photo on WhatsApp, I imagined you just like that, as sweet as your voice"; for others, the request to have the last conversation on video call "so you can see me", "so I can show you my house", testified to the desire to be seen in order to trustfully rely on a spacious container, capable of containing every aspect of the self in an integrated and durable way.

Notes

1 [R]apid changes have led to feelings of uncertainty and disorientation: changes in the sense of time (one could say that we suffer from the syndrome of haste, which implies a present without depth), but also in the sense of space (one is always connected, but at the same time distant and isolated); these aspects of neo-modernity influence today's psychology. (Castriota, 2020)

2 The French term *enveloppe* does not correspond exactly to the English term *envelope;* it may be considered a more nuanced version of the notion of container.

3 The case was treated by A. Fiori.

4 This sometimes manifested itself in the countertransference, loaded with bodily, sensory elements of the observer, who unconsciously became the bearer of split, unthinkable components projected onto him by the mother in crisis.

5 These considerations are, moreover, similar to what Fonagy and colleagues (Fonagy and Target, 1997) indicate regarding maternal "responsiveness" to the child.

6 The case was treated by I. Lapi.

7 The case was treated by L. Cresti.

8 The case was treated by L. Cresti.

9 The case was treated by E. Di Mauro.

10 The case was treated by C. Pratesi.

11 The case was treated by I. Lapi. A detailed description of Sonia's case can be found in Cresti and Lapi (1996).

12 In 2020, the AFPP set up a psychotherapeutic listening service from the earliest moments of the COVID-19 pandemic, offering online and telephone psychotherapeutic consultations for up to four interviews, and collaborated with the Ministry of Health on the second-level psychological support service.

13 Therapeutic consultations were open nationwide and users came from all over Italy. It was quite surprising that people often spoke to each other so far apart, in such different locations: this was very unusual for therapeutic work, which normally involves meetings between "neighbours" when conducted in person.

14 On the functions of the voice and its entanglement with the Unconscious, see also Pigozzi (2016).

15 The author is inspired by his own conception of music "as a sui generis language whose symbolic structure is isomorphic to that of our emotional and affective world". It is no coincidence that he dedicated his book "to the composers and musicians of all times who taught me how to hear words".

16 Mancia further states: A central role will be played in this process by the experiences the child has had in its endouterine growth. These experiences are all entrusted to sensoriality (primarily auditory but also somoesthetic, vestibular, gustatory), which will allow the foetus to perceive maternal rhythms (cardiac, respiratory, intestinal), its own rhythms and stimuli from the external environment. This will result in a maternal-fetal sensorimotor interaction whose essential characteristic is constancy and rhythmicity. These stimuli will function as 'model objects' for the formation of an initial outline of representations and will provide

the foetus with an ideal container for growth that is both physical and mental at the same time. (1998)

17 On the subject of the reassurance offered by the voice, we recall a well-known passage by Sigmund Freud, who tells of a child who was afraid of the dark and asked his aunt to talk to him because "if someone speaks there is light" (1905 [2001]); this passage is quoted in full in Chapter 9.

References

Anzieu, D. (1974). Le Moi-peau. *Nouvelle revue de psychanalyse: Le dehors et le dedans*, 9: 195–208.

Anzieu, D., Houzel, D., *et al.* (1987),. *Les enveloppes psychiques*. Paris: Dunod.

Bick, E. (1964). Notes on Infant Observation in Psychoanalytic Training. *International Journal of Psychoanalysis*, 45: 558–566.

Bion ,W. (1962). *Learning from Experience*. London: Karnac Books.

Bleger, J. (1967). *Simbiosis y ambigüedad*. Buenos Aires: Paidòs.

Brutti, C. and Brutti, R. (1996). Usi e abusi dell'Osservazione. *Quaderni di psicoterapia infantile*, 33.

Castriota, F. (2020). *Interpretare ascoltando. Atti della giornata scientifica SIEFPP*. Rome: Alpes.

Correale, A., Fadda, P., and Neri, C. (1994). *Letture bioniane*. Rome: Borla.

Cresti, L. (1997). *Therapeutic* Functions of Observing: A Reflection on the Containing Factors in *IO* and in Psychotherapy. Paper presented at The Infant Observation Conference, London (unpublished text).

Cresti, L. and Lapi, I. (1996). Dall'osservazione alla psicoterapia once-a-week. *Contrappunto*, 19: 15–28.

Ferrara Mori, G. (2001). Apprendere dall'osservazione. In L. Cresti, P. Farneti and C. Pratesi (eds), *Osservazione e trasformazione*. Rome: Borla.

Ferruta, A. (2012). Il silenzio è qualcuno che ascolta. Available at: www.spi-firenze.it/il-silenzio-e-qualcuno-che-ascolta-anna-ferruta/ (accessed 15 October 2020).

Fonagy, P. and Target, M. (1997). Attachment and Reflective Function: Their Role in Self-Organization. *Development and Psychopathology*, 9: 679–700.

Freud, S. (1905 [2001]). Three Essays on the Theory of Sexuality. In J. Strachey (ed.), *The Standard Edition of the Complete Psychological Works of Sigmund Freud*, vol. VII. London: Hogarth Press.

Haag, G. (1988). Réflections sur quelques jonctions psychotoniques et psychomotrices dans la première année de la vie. *Neuropsychiatrie de l'enfance et de l'adolescence*, 36(1): 36–52.

Harris, M. (1987). The Contribution of Observation of Mother-Infant Interaction and Development to the Equipment of a Psychoanalyst or Psychoanalytic Psychotherapist. In M. Harris and E. Bick, *Collected Papers of Martha Harris and Esther Bick*. London: Karnac Books.

Houzel, D. (1987). Le concept d'enveloppe psychique. In D. Anzieu, D. Houzel, *Les enveloppes psychiques*. Paris: Dunod.

Klein, M. (1952). Some Theoretical Conclusions Regarding the Emotional Life of the Infant. In P. Heimann, S. Isaacs, M. Klein and J. Riviere (eds), *Developments in Psychoanalysis*. London: Hogarth Press.

Mancia, M. (1998). *Riflessioni psicoanalitiche sul linguaggio musicale*. Bergamo: Moretti & Vitali Editori.

Mancia, M. (2004). *Sentire le parole*. Turin: Bollati Boringhieri.

Meltzer, D. (1967). *The Psychoanalytic Process*. London: Heinemann.

Ogden, T.H. (2016). *Reclaiming Unlived Life: Experiences in Psychoanalysis*. London: The British Psychoanalytical Society.

Pérez-Sánchez, M. (1982). *Observation de bébés*. Paris: Césura.

Pigozzi, L. (2016). *A nuda voce. Vocalità, inconscio, sessualità*. Bari: Poiesis.

Sabsay Foks, G. (1998). The voice: A psychoanalytic study. Available at: www.psy chomedia.it/neuro-amp/98-99-sem/sabsayfoks.html (accessed 15 March 2020).

Segal, H. (1957 [1984]). Note sulla formazione del simbolo. In *Scritti psicoanalitici*. Rome: Astrolabio.

Segal, H. (1981). *The Work of Hanna Segal: A Kleinian Approach to Clinical Practice*. Lanham, MD: Jason Aronson.

Winnicott, D.W. (1961). The Theory of the Infant-Parent Relationship. In D.W. Winnicott, *The Collected Works of D.W. Winnicott*, vol. 6, *1960–1963*. Oxford: Oxford University Press.

Winnicott, D.W. (1964 [1985]). L'importanza del setting nelle situazioni regressive in psicoanalisi. In *Esplorazioni psicoanalitiche*. Milan: Raffaello Cortina.

Winnicott, D.W. (1967 [1974]). La funzione di specchio della madre e della famiglia nello sviluppo infantile. In *Gioco e realtà*. Rome: Armand.

Chapter 3

The body in the therapeutic relationship

Luigia Cresti

Psychoanalysis has always recognised the importance of the body, but at the same time it has misunderstood its presence and role in treatment and the therapeutic relationship. There are many bodies, in fact, with which psychoanalysis has been concerned: from the erogenous body, the original biological seat of instinctual life (Freud's erogenous zones), to the body represented and fantasised in the unconscious (the good/bad breast, according to Klein, 1950). to the body felt as unity or non-integrated (Winnicott, 1970) and there is no doubt that the early sensations theorised in concepts such as Hoffer's Mouth-Ego (1950) or Spitz's primal cavity (1955) refer to the body. The psychoanalytic body, however, is a body that distances itself from the biological body of medicine, an inert object that can be broken down into organs, cells and functions: instead, it is a body that is subjectivised and sexualised from the outset, a body on which the first affective investments and anxieties of the human being are built (Carlini and Farneti, 1979). The phrase "body image" well expresses the symbolic value of the body:

> The body is the reassuring witness of the unity of the person, the object of the most immediate narcissistic contemplations ... the body is at the centre of all the moments of affective life ... There is no human activity of which the body is not the means and the aim, the instrument or the object.
>
> (Angelergues, 1964)

The body, therefore, is never neutral, but always felt, perceived and represented in a certain way, hated or loved: think of the difficulties in accepting one's own physicality, narcissistic disorders or more serious perceptual distortions, as in anorexia and bulimia.

Despite the fact that the body is a foundational element in ego-building processes, little attention has been paid by psychoanalysis to corporeality in the therapeutic relationship. Indeed, the most rigorous psychoanalytic approaches have focused mainly on the patient's words and verbal expressions, putting in second place the emotional signals sent directly from the patient's body and received, in the setting, in the therapist's bodily

DOI: 10.4324/9781032673721-4

countertransference. I would like to emphasise, however, as already noted in Chapter 2, the important role of the non-verbal communications that take place in the therapeutic interaction and that, before words or even independently of them, contribute to determining its course.[1] In non-verbal communications, it is body language, in its facial expressions, sound (infra-verbal) and gestural components that can convey important emotional messages and add significance to the therapeutic exchange. One could paraphrase the famous Freudian assertion "the Ego is first and foremost a body Ego" with the statement that "the psychotherapeutic relationship is first and foremost an encounter between two persons endowed with a body". In fact, after Freud and Breuer, a "mentalistic" preoccupation, so to speak, has been dominant in psychoanalysis in the sense that, in general, in the classical psychoanalytic session, bodies seem to have been considered almost accessories to mental processes. Some British psychoanalysts (Orbach, 2003; Fry, 2017)[2] have criticised the fact that in traditional psychoanalysis little attention has been paid to the body, the body as characterised by its own psychological and evolutionary history, while the mind has gained supremacy. An important change in perspective was introduced by the intersubjective current[3] and the attachment theory, which emphasised the central importance of the relationship with the external object, even in its physical reality; a significant contribution was permitted more clearly by observational methodologies: Infant Research[4] and, above all, Infant Observation, according to Esther Bick, have made it possible to grasp the close interconnection between bodily experiences and mental processes from the very beginning, and have helped us, even in therapeutic work with adults, to approach the earliest and deepest levels of emotional experience, precisely from the facts of the body.

An interesting aspect of this critical, intersubjective rethinking of the role of the body in therapy is the observation that in traditional psychoanalysis little attention has been paid to the patient's body, but even less to that of the therapist. In fact, according to Orbach (2003). the therapist's way of "being in the body" can influence the patient's feelings about his or her own body, initiating a pathway to help him or her find a personal "embodiment"; the therapist, therefore, must pose the problem of bringing his or her own soma into the relationship with the patient, as well as paying attention to those countertransference resonances at the body level that the patient may induce. With regard to the importance of the countertransference sensations experienced on a somatic level by the therapist, Orbach describes cases in which they appear to be visceral translations of the patient's primitive experiences; in short, it can be hypothesised that our countertransference, even in its bodily aspects, can open up great opportunities for understanding and treatment.

The rediscovery of the body in Italian psychoanalysis

The above-mentioned criticisms made by the English psychoanalysts do not take into account that, in fact, in contemporary Italian psychoanalysis there is a tendency to reconsider in a new light the importance of the body in psychic development and in the clinic. In this regard, the concept, proposed by Lemma, of *embodied setting* appears of particular interest and originality, to indicate how "the physical appearance and presence of the analyst and his or her sensoriality provide a form of 'embodied' containment, such that any change on the physical level can mobilise certain anxieties and fantasies in the patient" (2019).

She emphasises how:

> the containment provided by the analyst's physical appearance, the way he "inhabits" his body and the physical space of the room are felt in the same way as the other environmental elements of the setting: the way he breathes, the way he sits, the nods of assent, the way he gets up at the end of the session ... become expected elements of the context.
>
> (Lemma, 2019)

Lemma takes from Bleger (1967) the concept of "symbiotic transference", typical of those patients who need to relate to the therapist's body as an invariant part of the setting, as if it were one with the environment: any change in the analyst's somatic level, since it marks separation from him, creates intense anxiety in the patient and reveals his "phantom world", which also reverberates in the therapist's countertransference. Along a similar line of thought also moves C. Bronstein (2017), who considers the setting as an element that can evoke even pre-symbolic fantasies, through the patient's experience of sharing a physical space with the analyst and through his bodily presence.

Another aspect worth exploring is the relationship the therapist has with his or her own body:

> one has to know something of our experience of *being-in-a-body* and of being, inevitably, the object of the other's gaze ... As analysts we have to be aware that our body continually communicates something of how we feel about ourselves and what we think about patients.
>
> (Lemma, 2019)

This dimension is particularly important when working with patients who are unable to feel at home in their own bodies because often, without knowing it, "they look at how others inhabit their bodies to see what is possible ... the analyst's body is perceived as libidinally invested ..." (Lemma, 2019).

At the same time, Lemma develops a reflection on somatic countertransference, starting from the assumption that the way in which we "listen" to the patient's body and its narrative is filtered by the therapist's subjectivity, which includes bodily and psychic components; the analyst's somatic countertransference should therefore be considered a fundamental aspect of his or her internal setting.

Brosio, too, laments that the area of the implicit mode of communication that takes place between the therapist's body and the patient's body is still unexplored:

> Today, the body as such is increasingly theorised, but the accounts of the two bodies in the analysis room and the mutual impact of one on the other are still under-represented. The body is an inescapable tool in human relations because of its extraordinary communicative potential; inter-subjectivity is first and foremost inter-corporeity, the encounter is first and foremost an encounter of bodies. But if it is true that in patients with a deficit at the level of self-organisation, the observation of the analyst's real embodied body is vital for their evolution, why maintain a set-up that foresees, with the use of the couch, the "out-of-scope" of the analyst's body? Perhaps we need to prepare ourselves for some displacement in our comfortable analysis room?
>
> (2019)

An interesting contribution to the discussion on these issues was recently made by S. Bolognini (2020) during the debate held in Rome, L'Ascolto Psicoanalitico [Listening Psychoanalytically] on the occasion of a meeting of the Italian Section of EFPP in 2020. Starting from the appreciation of an unusual vision of the "biology of psychotherapy" – proposed by M. Biondi (2020) who alludes to the psycho-corporeal interchange between patient and therapist – Bolognini criticised the radical positions of those psychoanalytic schools that have overestimated the importance of representation as the only functional factor to be considered in psychotherapy:

> Representation is undoubtedly a fundamental level of psychic functioning and psychoanalysis; but to consider *it* psychoanalysis *tout court* ... makes one lose sight of a more complex and articulated conception of the human being ... There exists in place a psycho-sensory and psycho-corporeal reality, which can use the instrument of metaphor and equivalence: that is, something experiential that allows us to feel how psychic states are equivalent to bodily states, or bodily events or bodily processes ... During sessions we can feel operating, far beyond our conscious technical intentions, these processes that take place in continuity between the corporeal and the psychic.

Exponents of Analytical Field Theory (in Italy, Ferro, Civitarese and others) have also emphasised the presence of the body in patient-analyst communication; as Civitarese states:

> There is never only a symbolic exchange. Words are always used also in their signifier value, they always contribute to generating the material

environment in which the analysis takes place, but sometimes they exert a pressure that is so intense as to become almost *physical*, like being touched, caressed, pushed or cradled concretely. With one patient several times I had to restrain myself from literally plugging my ears, as if the words were sticking in me. On other occasions I experienced symptoms of cardiac neurosis because of the tension that was being created.

(2013)

In this "somatic field", the analyst resorts to the use of bodily rêverie, a function capable of grasping the most primitive levels of communication. For Civitarese, bodily rêverie, which is particularly useful in reaching patients with serious deficiencies in symbolic capacity, is placed at the first link of the chain, until it gradually arrives at an interpretation with an increasingly complex integration of thought.

Clinical experience

We too have verified, on the basis of our clinical experience, the significant role that the body can play in the therapeutic relationship: that of the patient, first of all, but also that of the therapist. That is to say, on the one hand, it is important to pay attention to the non-verbal messages that patients unconsciously transmit with their body (mimicry, posture, overall physical appearance, the pleasantness or otherwise of his appearance, body smells, etc.); on the other hand, it is also fundamental to pay attention to our physical (countertransference) sensations that can be indicators of significant aspects, non-verbalised and non-verbalisable, that the patient projects onto us.

In short, it is a matter of reconsidering the meanings conveyed by the bodily manifestations and the sense-perceptions of both patient and therapist. These aspects are particularly pregnant in the face-to-face setting, where the non-verbal assumes a pre-eminent function in activating and transmitting the transference and countertransference messages, through a real "body to body", as underlined by Bolognini.

I would like to refer here to my personal clinical experience, which can partly illustrate these concepts: in some situations of treatment of female patients, in a face-to-face setting, an important role in the development of the case seems to have been played not only by the containing framework of a regular setting and by the cognitive-interpretive communication provided verbally by the therapist, but also by the *interactive emotional communication* made possible by the face-to-face setting and mediated by multiple, subtle bodily channels. I believe that with these patients, who presented a perturbation in their feminine identity in various respects, the more direct relationship made possible by the face-to-face setting implicitly offered a sort of model for the affects: the therapist's emotional reactions and profound experiences regarding central themes of femininity, touched upon by the patients (the relationship with the mother, both internal and external, the relationship with the body, as sexualized, the desires and fears connected with love relationships, the feelings and fantasies about pregnancy and motherhood), even if not verbally communicated by the therapist, were probably registered by the patients, who integrated them to some extent within themselves, as a trace for a greater definition of their female identity.

It can be important, in short, for a patient to see, to perceptively grasp aspects, albeit minimal, of the therapist's non-verbal attitude, which convey the quality of her emotional resonance and, at the same time, the sense of her own body, of her own person.

It can therefore be assumed that in the course of a psychoanalytic psychotherapy in a face-to-face setting, sensations, affects, significant identifying impulses can be activated from the *mutual perception* and *sensory contact of the patient with the non-verbal expression of the therapist*, reflecting the impact of his or her participation, but also the deep and personal sense of self that the therapist possesses. This hypothesis is consistent with Winnicott's statement that "the patient needs the reality of the analyst's emotions in order to feel the reality of his own person" (1947). With regard, then, to the patient's body, it is important to pay attention to the unconsciously communicative meaning that mimic and postural signs and "gestures in the body" (Guerrini, 2020) may have, but at the same time to take into consideration the patient's physical development history and the subjective sense he /she has of his /her own body, bearing in mind how the somatic element is fundamental in the construction and definition of the Self. One must also consider the suggestion, particularly appropriate in child therapy, that "when the patient needs support offered to his or her primitive needs, mental and emotional containment cannot be separated from the more corporeal feeling of being held" (Fry, 2017).

The following cases broaden our reflection on the importance of the body in psychotherapy, in those particular situations of suffering linked to the body image and when the physical conditions of the patient or therapist become overwhelmingly evident: the patient's disability and the therapist's bodily modifications, in this case, of her pregnancy.

Anita: a body you don't like
Esmeralda Di Mauro

Anita is a 20-year-old girl who comes to therapy because of her difficulties in managing relationships: she suddenly shifts from idealisation to devaluation and thus is unable to build lasting relationships. Her encounter with a boy in whom she begins to have a sincere interest gives her the impetus to ask for help; she fears that she will put the aforementioned dynamics into action with him and, consequently, lose him. In the first session she tells me that she would have preferred a male therapist. It soon emerges how Anita manages to invest much more in phallic aspects rather than in feminine ones (women are, in fact, always devalued in her imagination), a sensitive issue being body image and the low libidinal investments made in it. Tall, thin, with a pronounced nose, nothing in her enhances her femininity. She looks like a young child, still uncertain whether to be a boy or a girl.

Her identity is undefined, the representation of the bodily self is markedly depressive (she often dresses in dark colours and appears neglected). The body seems to be experienced as fragile and insubstantial; it will emerge later in the course of therapy how it has been invested, by the parents, exclusively as an object of medical care (both father and mother work in the health sector and the patient has never had either a paediatrician or, subsequently, a general practitioner). One may think that her body, rather than being an object of tenderness and mystery, has been an object of control.

Throughout the first period of therapy, I found it difficult to address the patient as an adult as I experienced her as a child. The defence consistently put in place was inhibition: hardly any drive or emotional movements were observed, the sessions often took place in a flat, calm atmosphere and I felt I had to move slowly, gently, and that what was important was to be genuinely there, to provide the patient with the possibility of a protected relationship, to let myself be observed. One can think that in the patient there was a difficulty in identifying herself as a woman: she did not like her body, especially her legs which she saw as "crooked" and her breasts which she saw as "big" (again a devaluation of the feminine and fear of emerging libidinal drives). In this sense, the possibility of carrying out sessions face-to-face, observing me, identifying with me, imagining me and reading through my body her pleasure was one of the transformative elements of the therapy.

In a spontaneous joke during a session, I told her, "I'll have to be careful how I dress!" (the patient was talking about the devaluations of her friends' way of dressing), the patient smiled at me: in that sentence there was the story of our relationship, the relationship between our bodies, our way of being women. We can read in this sentence an underlining of the aspects of caring for oneself and for the other, a bringing into play of the body with its clothes, its infinite possibilities of being, its drives; it means saying to each other: "We are here, we observe each other, we take care of each other, I am waiting for you, I take care of me while waiting, I take care of you also through taking care of me ...".

I thought, from the beginning, that the patient was looking for a woman (a substitute for the mother figure) in the therapeutic pathway to use as a model to grow:

> You know, I'm a curious person and sometimes I ask myself: I wonder what she thinks ... I fantasise, I think she's a very serene person, this she tells me, that she has a good private life, a boyfriend, otherwise she couldn't tell me the things she says! She's certainly very busy ... and she really enjoys her work, you can see that ... I wonder how old she is, how long she's been working, how she felt with her first patient ... I wonder if

her private life influences her work, I mean, what she says will also depend on her private life! I wonder if she likes animals, if she lives alone ... I think she's a beautiful woman, she looks like Vittoria Belvedere [a beautiful Italian actress, whose surname also means "good-looking"]. She takes care in her clothing and pays attention to the combinations. I think, that Great Woman!

It is interesting, in my opinion, to observe how much the words uttered by the patient have to do with the libidinal dimension, with the pleasure she could observe in her relationship with me (the pleasure linked to work is also linked to the pleasure of the relationship with her). The identification (Belvedere) is with the therapist's body (perceived as well dressed) which can inhabit libidinal impulses (boyfriend) and perhaps can also solicit them in her ("Great Woman", an expression not only of idealisation but also of falling in love with). Meanwhile, Anita begins to show more of her femininity, to "inhabit her body", to take care of her "intimate" underwear.

After about a year, during a session in which the topic is our relationship, she tells me that she often fantasises about me, she likes to imagine me:

> You look a lot like Vittoria Belvedere, I guess you live in Bellosguardo [the name of an area near Florence, which also means "beautiful to look at"] ... I fantasise about how she might feel about me ... We kind of look alike ...

The body in disability
Isabella Lapi

When the patient is ill or disabled, the therapist's body is particularly brought into play and is charged with specific therapeutic values. In these cases, the patient's body overbearingly demands to be seen, felt and accepted, even before being understood, and it is from the corporeal that the therapist must start in order to get to the mental; vice versa, to use thought and, with it, interpretations right away would risk speaking only to the more evolved areas of the mind, creating a pseudo-therapeutic process that does not rest on mind-body integration but deepens its dissociation. It is crucial, instead "to encourage in the first instance a progressive approach to the perception of the body and its sensations in order to build an initial framework of the subject's identity"(Lombardi, 2003).

To do this, the therapist often finds herself using her own bodily perceptions, captured not only through her own bodily countertransference reactions but also through an identificatory movement: a kind of bodily empathy is thus created that allows the patient to feel truly understood by a therapist who is on her side, both are at the same starting point to embark together on a journey of thought and understanding.

Anna: The need for bodily empathy

Anna is a young woman who has been blind since birth; she has quickly achieved a high degree of autonomy in life but in a condition of profound relational loneliness. She had been in psychotherapy for almost a year for depression when the lockdown caused by the pandemic forced the psychotherapist to interrupt the in-person sessions. Anna, while understanding this, suffers greatly, and the replacement of the session with two weekly phone calls, suggested by the therapist, is not enough to fill her sense of lack. What she misses is the sensory contact with the therapist:

> I miss coming to the office, walking through the neighbourhood with its sounds and smells and then ringing the doorbell … her greeting me warmly at the door, giving me her arm … I sit and she looks at me while I talk, I can't see her but I feel her gaze on me, this helps me.

This sensory emptiness reminds her of the affective void Anna feels inside, rooted in her first, unhappy, childhood experiences; she asks for the therapist's arm to enter the therapy room even though she knows very well how to move in space with a cane: she needs bodily contact that makes her feel the presence of a loving, helping Other, seeing and accepting her fragile childish side, which has remained hidden and unseen inside the independent and strong woman. The warmth of the greeting and the therapist's gaze on her convey acceptance and containment, and that sense of existence that the "joyful" mother conveys to her baby when she looks at it, happy that it is there (Vallino and Macciò, 2010).

In her relationship with the therapist, Anna regressed to the early infant state whose needs could not be met by her mother, who withdrew from her relationship with her upon her birth, plunging her into severe depression and forcing Anna to quickly gain independence.

The therapist is profoundly affected by the sensory emptiness of the patient's disability, and tries to perceive it with her own body by imagining the world in the dark, sometimes even trying to close her eyes, only to reopen them immediately afterwards, feeling disturbed. Above all, she feels resounding within herself the desperate affective emptiness of that new-born child, unseen by her mother, because she is too difficult to love, due to her disability. Spontaneously, the therapist responds, in an adult and respectful manner, to that deprivation of sensory and affective relations, making available, before her own words, her own sensoriality, so Anna is helped to recover and integrate into her Self those fragile infantile parts, long split off and denied.

The therapist's pregnancy
Giulia Mercuriali

The therapist's pregnancy represents one of those conditions in which the theme of the body becomes most evident in psychotherapeutic work, and the therapist's physical condition means that her soma enters consistently into the relationship with the patient. The *real* baby in the therapist's body represents a real irruption into the therapeutic space, it is an inescapable fact of reality with which both patient and therapist have to come to terms.

The therapist's pregnancy, especially when working with children, implies major reorganisations and leads to the need to reorganise the identity and relational plane so that a real and imaginary *third party* enters the therapeutic field. S. Fenster illustrated how the therapist's body during pregnancy follows its own rules with a "concrete, irreversible and strongly evocative violation of the setting" (Fenster et al., 1986). Modifications of the setting and of the relationship take shape that deserve further study, in that the therapist's body becomes the object of identifications and projections, an instrument through which the patient finds himself relating to a therapist who is not the one he knows and with whom he measures himself during the course of the sessions.

We report on the difficulties a therapist faced during her first pregnancy, with respect to her psychotherapeutic engagement with Carolina, a 12-year-old girl in foster care whom she had been following for some time.

Carolina: the body, emotional resonance and communication

The therapist reported that she had many uncertainties about how and when to tell Carolina the news of her pregnancy. Her body, together with the way she dressed, did not yet clearly show her growing belly and allowed the therapist to dwell in this uncertainty. A consequence of the pregnancy, which the therapist had not perceived before, was that she became aware of how both her mind and the way she attuned herself and her patients were changing. With Carolina, the situation was particularly delicate since the girl had been placed with another family by her birth family; moreover, the same biological family had quite recently had another daughter who had been allowed to stay with them instead.

"I had decided that this was the session in which I would communicate about my expectation but still something inside me made me hesitate," the therapist notes. She had waited for the morphological ultrasound scan to tell her patients about the pregnancy; the ultrasound scan was elected as the moment when, in relation to the knowledge derived from the physical and structural investigation of the foetus, even of its tiny body in formation, it was given a name and began to really exist; from that moment on, that "something" growing in the body could also be shared.

The therapist's body came to be the powerful medium that allowed this growth, the fertile ground for the baby that was growing inside her, but also the external structure that would be connected with the risk (associated with increased emotional and psychological vulnerability) of transference reactions intertwined with themes of separation, loss, abandonment, jealousy, sibling rivalry, sexuality, oedipal issues and envy.

The young patient arrived at the session and, after the initial greetings, the child Tommaso suddenly appeared on the scene: the patient was talking about a cousin of hers with whom she had come into conflict, but the name was the same as the one the therapist had chosen for the baby she was carrying! Tommaso was the patient's cousin and part of the foster family; he was described as the little one of the family, loved even though he was bound to the foster parents by a complex and intricate relationship. Carolina and Tommaso often played together and she was happy to spend time with him; beyond affection, however, she experienced him as intrusive and observed how he forced everyone to listen only to his needs: "He's like a little brother, but he's also a nuisance."

The therapist found herself thinking about how her own Tommaso would also "break" something: the continuity of the work and the security that no one else would occupy her therapist's mind during their sessions, on resumption. The therapist then found herself having to explore this narrative with the girl and communicate her pregnancy to her. The body and its changes, even if not communicated, had nevertheless conveyed the emotional and transference connection of the patient who had never, in the previous years of therapy, brought "her" own Tommaso into the room.

In the session, Carolina now introduced a character that opened up the possibility of vivifying, actualising what was happening in the mind and body of the therapist and consequently in the therapeutic field: a presence that allowed the narration of conflict, jealousy and mystery on which it was possible to reflect without the risk of feeling expelled or abandoned.

The body functioned as a powerful means of non-verbal communication, fostering an emotional resonance in the relationship.

Beatrice: between physical distance and emotional closeness

In another case that I treated during my pregnancy (Beatrice, a 27-year-old girl), therapy proceeded slowly due to the general situation triggered by the COVID-19 pandemic that started in 2020. In those first months, it was difficult for the therapists to cope with the physical distance resulting from the need to carry on with online therapy.

Therapist and patient were no longer sharing the same room and therefore, in this case, the growing belly and the change in the body of the therapist, who had not yet communicated her pregnancy, were not visible. But this burst into a dream that Beatrice brought into the session: the patient, a medical student, was in a hospital delivery room; she was assisting a friend, an acquaintance whom she held in high esteem but did not feel close to, to deliver her baby. She wondered why her partner was not there to assist her, but the fact that she was chosen by her friend still pleased her. At a certain point, just as the pains were getting worse and the moment of delivery was approaching, it was the patient herself who took the place of the birthing woman: it was she who gave birth to a baby boy, tiny but healthy.

The therapist was struck by this "substitution", which occurred just some time before her baby was born. She then realised how, in spite of the patient's initial criticism of having to meet at a distance, the work had nevertheless allowed her to deal with separation issues without feeling abandoned: the possibility of being able to accept and realise that she had to rely on her own resources to be born came to light. Through this dream, it was possible for Beatrice to begin to feel supportive of herself and also become "pregnant" with good things.

Conclusion

Our clinical experience therefore converges, in many respects, with certain positions of contemporary psychoanalysis; with regard to our reflection on the theme of the body in psychotherapy, the central aspects that in our opinion are particularly relevant are:

- the value of the therapist's flesh-and-blood presence in the session: we have acknowledged the importance of the face-to-face setting which allows a communicative use of the non-verbal bodily messages, in a more consistent manner than can occur with the couch (we have already described, for instance, how, among the non-interpretive therapeutic factors, the visual *enveloppe* function offered by the therapist is important);
- the communicative meaning that the patient's bodily manifestations can have through the various channels of expression;
- attention to the therapist's bodily reactions/responses to the contents brought by the patient; understanding these can contribute to the unfolding of the therapeutic function;
- greater consideration of "bodily actions", i.e., the therapist's "talking" actions and micro-actions (shaking hands, responding to being touched by the patient, gestures etc.). as we will describe in Chapter 4.

Notes

1 See, for example, the multiple implications of looks and sound messages.
2 S. Orbach founded The Women's Therapy Centre in London and New York; she was columnist for *The Guardian* newspaper.
3 This current of thought that originated in the United States has also influenced psychoanalytic reflection here; a central aspect of it is the belief that the intrapsychic is determined by the relationship between people, and that psychoanalysis is *interaction*. Cf. Panizza (2008).
4 Infant Research shows how the intrapsychic dimension is constructed from the relationship. To understand the intertwining of Infant Research, Infant Observation and psychoanalysis, see Vallino and Macciò (2012).

References

Angelergues, R. (1964). Le corps et ses images. *Evolution Psychiatrique*, 29(2): 181–216.

Biondi, M. (2020). Biologia della psicoterapia. In SIEFPP, *L'ascolto psicoanalitico*. Rome: Alpes.

Bleger, J. (1967). *Simbiosis y ambiguedad, e studio psicoanalitico*. Buenos Aires: Editorial Paidòs.

Bolognini, S. (2020). L'ascolto psicoanalitico. In SIEFPP, *L'ascolto psicoanalitico*. Rome: Alpes.

Bronstein, C. (2017). The Unconscious Fantasy in Sessions: Recognising Its Form. *The International Psychoanalytic Annals*, 9: 65–87.

Brosio, C. (2019). Abitare il corpo. *Rivista di Psicoanalisi*, LXV(1): 147–155.

Carlini, M.G. and Farneti, P. (1979). *Il corpo in psicologia*. Bologne: Pàtron.

Civitarese, G. (2013). Campo incarnato, rêverie corporea e pazienti con blocchi della simbolizzazione. *Educazione Sentimentale*, 20: 25–31.

Fenster, S., Phillips, B.S., Estelle, R.G., and Rapaport, E.R.G. (1986). *The Therapist's Pregnancy: Intrusion into the Analytic Space*. London: Routledge.

Fry, C. (2017). Some Reflections on the Problem of Narcissism in Psychoanalytic Practice. In V. Hunter (ed.), *Psicoanalisti in azione*. Rome: Astrolabio.

Guerrini, B. (2020). Rappresentazioni in azione. Stati non rappresentati della mente e potenzialità figurativa del dispositivo analitico. AFPP (unpublished text).

Hoffer, W. (1950). Development of Body-Ego. *The Psychoanalytic Study of the Child*, 5: 18–23.

Klein, M. (1950). *The Psychoanalysis of Children*. London: The Hogarth Press.

Lemma, A. (2019). Il legame estetico: l'uso del corpo dell'analista e del corpo della stanza di analisi da parte del paziente. *Rivista di psicoanalisi*, LXV(1): 107–127.

Lombardi, R. (2003). Alterità del corpo, conflittualità, identità. *Interazioni*, 2: 84–96.

Orbach, S. (2003). There Is No Such Thing as a Body. *British Journal of Psychotherapy*, 20(1): 3–15.

Spitz, R. (1955). The Primal Cavity: A Contribution to the Genesis of Perception and Its Role for Psychoanalytic Theory. *The Psychoanalytic Study of the Child*, 10: 215–240.

Vallino, D. and Macciò, M. (2010). *Essere neonati*. Rome: Borla.

Winnicott, D.W. (1947). Hate in the Counter-Transference. *International Journal of Psychoanalysis*, 30: 69–74.

Winnicott, D.W. (1970). On the Basis of Self in the Body. In D.W. Winnicott, *Psychoanalytic Explorations*. London: Routledge.

Chapter 4

Gestures that touch, actions that heal

Isabella Lapi

Beyond words, there is a *body talk* that enters the psychotherapy room and helps to define the relationship and the therapeutic process. It is the non-verbal and pre-verbal language of gestures and actions that belongs to all of us, and which refers directly to the primary experience of relationship with the mother, within whose body and mind life is formed. The mother-child relationship begins as a bodily relationship from the moment of conception, when the egg and the foetus need the mother's body to survive and grow, and continues after birth, when the mother nourishes with her breast, caresses and cradles, transmitting love and joy for the child's existence, and consoles with her arms and the sound of her voice when she feels the baby's pain and anguish. The baby expresses with the body needs and emotions that the mother feels, in turn, with the body ... eyes, touch, guts ... understands them through a bodily resonance that activates thought and triggers the process of mental transformation; words will then come between them. The mother cares for the child through the rêverie function, which is a mental function but is also, and even before that, a bodily rêverie. This primordial experience of communication remains in our internal world and recurs in adult relationships and, of course, in the therapeutic relationship.

The language of gestures and actions is of fundamental importance as a vehicle of conscious and unconscious contents on the part of the patient and the therapist and finds its place in psychotherapy alongside the verbal language of free associations, dreams and interpretations. If recognised and well used, gestures and actions become healing.

From *agieren* to *InterpretAction*, a long journey

The early Freud touched patients, but then the gesture and its communicative meanings were long lost in psychoanalysis. Freud interpreted the patient's actions outside and inside the session as putting acting in place of remembering, attributing to these acts the meaning of resistance: "It is most undesirable for us that the patient, outside of transference, should act rather than remember" (Freud, 1938 [2001]). It was a very important element in the

DOI: 10.4324/9781032673721-5

development of psychoanalysis (Etchegoyen, 1986) to have identified the "agieren" (Freud, 1938 [2001]) as a way of not thinking about the repressed elements by acting them both in and out and thus attacking the analytic work, with the corollary that the analyst also had to be very careful not to act in turn by yielding to the pressure of the patient's actions on him. Considering enactments as an error to be avoided at all times, while maintaining the utmost abstinence and neutrality, undoubtedly helped to avoid errors but, in time, led to demonising enactments as such dangerous material that its communicative significance and the therapeutic advantages to be gained from it were underestimated. In communicating with the patient, the consequence was to privilege verbal language, while non-verbal language for a very long time was seen, at most, as performing "a function of support, of complement, of substitution, of reversal, which not infrequently proves essential, but with the aim of translating all this as soon as possible into verbal language" (Mori, 1993).

Over time, alongside this classical position, now recognised by all as excessively rigid and simplified, a line of thought has developed in psychoanalysis that has attenuated the opposition between acting and thinking in order to recognise the transformative importance also of "acted" behaviour with respect to "verbalised" behaviour (Guerrini Degli Innocenti, 2017). This change is directly linked to the evolution of the paradigms of psychoanalysis, also prompted by the changes in the clinic; we merely mention them, referring their in-depth study to the contemporary literature by now copious:[1] the recognition of projective identification as an instrument of communication; the shift from the focus on countertransference to the acknowledgement of the therapist as an interacting subject, hence the relational turn and the intersubjective conceptions of analysis; the use of the concept of enactment that sheds new light on acting; the diffusion of the theory of the analytical field; the discovery of the interpsychic flow; the new conception of the unrepressed unconscious. These and other passages indicate that attention has shifted to the communicative process that develops in analysis and psychotherapy, and that gestures and actions have been legitimised in their function of transmitting messages beyond verbal symbolic representation, thus discovering new ways of accessing the patient's deepest contents. On a technical level, a new perspective opens up, aimed at the identification and implementation of technical tools other than the classical ones. As A.M. Nicolò has recently stated, psychoanalytic technique itself is in fact changing: non-symbolised psychic contents find modes of expression other than verbal symbolic representation and can only be observed, understood and communicated in the action and bodily interaction of the couple; it follows that interpretation loses its absolute primacy in favour of other instruments of treatment that pertain to action, "which mobilise the analyst as a person and as a new object in the relationship" (2019). In this changed context, even enactment, once considered almost a "bump in the road", is now recognised in its therapeutic value that makes it a major analytical tool.

We owe to T. Jacobs (1986; 2001) the definition of enactment, a mediating concept in this evolution of the technique. For Jacobs, enactments are behaviours, either of the analyst or the patient or both, related to the transference-countertransference interaction in response to emerging fantasies and conflicts. If they are not recognised by the therapist, they are repressed but continue to exert a destructive action on the analysis: collusion with the patient, narcissistic defence of one's own self-esteem, manipulation of the patient towards certain topics and towards the analyst's point of view, and so on. Enactments bring therapeutic work to a standstill, negative therapeutic resistance and impasses, and must be correctly managed with interpretation: only in this way, coming out of the meaning of a blind "agieren" as opposed to thinking, can they be of great help in dealing with deep conflicts that have remained obscured up to that moment, and reactivate the therapeutic process. Indeed, enactments always reveal contents of the utmost importance and become valuable tools for dealing with aspects that would otherwise remain inaccessible.[2]

An original and decisive impetus to the technical breakthrough that recognised the therapeutic value of the therapist's actions in the session was given by T.H. Ogden, who introduced the concept of "interpretive action" or "interpretation-in-action": "communication of the analyst's understanding of the transference-countertransference to the analysand through an activity rather than a symbolic verbalization" (Ogden, 1994).

The leap that Ogden makes consists no longer in merely examining the impact of the analyst's actions on the patient and on the relationship in order to use it in the verbal interpretation, but rather in enacting actions that become a real "interpretive vehicle" (Ogden, 1994).

Similar results have been achieved by the French school: R. Prat and P. Israel (2013). for example, use the term *InterpretAction* to designate those relational acts of the therapist that introduce linguistic and behavioural acts into the interpretive function of analysis. The impact of this work of the analyst between word and action has a strong transformative power as "repetition of the processes at the very origin of the construction of psychism" (Prat, 2009).

The work with seriously ill patients and the constant change of pathology towards states where the symbolic defect and the deficiency of the internal container prevail[3] undoubtedly prompted the search for new therapeutic tools that would make these patients accessible to analytic work. These are patients who use projective identification as a fundamental mode of communication and defence, and their failure to "put into words" testifies to an early dysfunction in the processes of psyche-soma integration, created from the first interactive exchanges with the mother. With them, instead of the exchange of words on which psychoanalytic treatment is usually based, it is necessary to use acted exchanges and manifestations that involve the body and draw on the most primitive communicative modes of the primary relationship. Understanding and internalising verbal interpretations would be very difficult and would produce greater distance; the therapist, especially in the early stages of treatment, can only reach them through the enactment of a thought, feeling or fantasy.

Racamier's (1997) work in therapeutic communities for psychotics makes this different way of interpreting particularly clear. With a strategy devised and defined by the treatment team, "speaking objects" and "speaking actions" are chosen for each patient, i.e., concrete objects and concrete actions that act as a transitional area between external and internal reality. This strategy translates the symbol into concrete representation and the thought into action in order to be able to transmit it in a way that can be assimilated by the patient and to promote its integration into his psyche.[4] This strategy, very widespread in therapeutic communities, is also used in individual psychotherapy in order to facilitate the start of the relationship and the creation of the intermediate area of play (Winnicott, 1971). For example, in therapy with children and adolescents, the therapist may allow the child to take home an object from the room or, not considering it appropriate to resort to interpretation, may give or lend an object that can concretely transmit the desired symbolic message.

Actually, experiences with serious patients have highlighted phenomena and functions that belong to therapeutic work in any case, with any kind of patient, especially in some particular moments such as impasses, situations of intense emotional burden, or when speech is used defensively and the patient can only be reached with direct emotional experience.

Communicating on another level

The interpsychic flow identified by S. Bolognini (2019) allows a better understanding of how this direct emotional experience can take place in the session with profoundly transformative effects. When the verbal interpretation, which addresses the conscious ego, does not prove adequate for the patient's possibilities to accept it, or there is a need for more direct and intense communication, other communicative levels succeed in immediately transmitting the therapeutic response to his internal difficulty, such as the interpsychic level, which joins the intrapsychic and intersubjective as a new level of therapeutic action.

The interpsychic is that "functional level of high permeability shared between two psychic apparatuses" that skips the interpretive talk to get directly to the internal world (Bolognini, 2019). In the interpsychic communicative flow, the two internal worlds of analyst and patient come into intimate contact, transmitting contents that directly reach the patient's preconscious, bypassing the defensive ego and the superego (a metaphor for this is the cat flap, that little door that allows the cat to enter and exit autonomously without having to call on its owner to open the main door). Rising from the pre-conscious, the interpsychic flow appears in moments of intense and profound communication, spontaneous and rather rare, requiring a good attunement of the analyst first of all with himself, and then with the internal world and the dynamic organisation of the patient, so that it is possible to transmit combined verbal-sensory elements from within the analyst to within the patient.

(Bolognini, 2008)

The relief they bring to both members of the therapeutic couple is immediate, thanks to the content they convey, which touches on deep themes of conflict and the patient's object and transference relationships, but also thanks to them feeling together that the therapeutic relationship is alive and authentic, that therapist and patient are united in a communion of purpose and mind, in a "temporary and transient condition of shared and cooperative fusionality" (Bolognini, 2008). The interpsychic is expressed in acts and words that are often very simple in appearance, but which imply a psychic process of great complexity.

Franca: the promise of the fairy tale

Franca's[5] initial sessions in psychotherapy for depression are characterised by long silences, which shatter the discourse and make any attempt at interpretation fall on deaf ears. One day, Franca breaks the silence and says that she is glad to hear her mother on the phone; the therapist asks her what they talk about and Franca replies that they talk about trivial, everyday things. At the therapist's comment about the need to have her mother beside her in order to feel protected, Franca nods mechanically and closes herself in silence again, keeping her eyes downcast for a long time. Then suddenly she says: "See, doctor, I have no arguments to speak about, you tell me something." The therapist replies: "Maybe a fairy tale!" Franca, surprised, looks brightly at the therapist and then they both open up in a spontaneous smile. At the end of the session, Franca says that she will phone her mother more often.

For Franca, it is not the things she and her mother say to each other that count, but the fact that they hear each other over the phone, so it is not the therapist's interpretative comments that reach her, but the fairy tale that the therapist is willing to tell. The fairy tale encloses, as in a casket, the recognition of Franca's regressive needs and the unexpressed feelings of transference/countertransference: it is not important to open this casket at once and name its contents one by one; what matters now is knowing it is there. Franca and the therapist welcome it with relief: contact and hope start to appear, words will come later.

In therapeutic consultation and in psychotherapy with children, the "cat flap" of the interpsychic flow is the game, especially in its narrative dimension that allows the child to narrate his experience, to give it order and meaning, helped in this by the therapist, not with saturated interpretations, but with the co-construction of the game. The therapist allows himself to be involved in the game, uses his own empathic feeling towards the characters of the internal world staged by the child, and actively participates in the story told. In this way of working, well known to childhood therapists, in which the therapist intentionally disposes himself to suspend the use of interpretation, we can see the choice to place himself at the level of the interpsychic flow and dialogue with the child by speaking to his preconscious.

Emma: the fear of Little Red Riding Hood

Emma's[6] father asked for help for 6-year-old Emma, because following her father's illness which led to fears of a heart attack, Emma began to manifest a series of intense fears. The father is the only parent the child can really rely on, as the mother has a serious psychiatric disorder. At the new meeting with the therapist, Emma arrives very sad and silent, looks expectantly at the therapist, who immediately proposes: "Shall we play?" As if revived, Emma takes the puppets and sets up the story of Little Red Riding Hood who asks her Queen Mother and King Father for permission to go to visit her grandmother to get biscuits and in the woods meets the Wolf. The therapist, to whom the character of the Wolf is entrusted, says in a threatening voice: "Now I'm going to scare you, I'm going to eat Grandma, and then Father King and Mother Queen...". Little Red Riding Hood rebels: "I am not afraid of you, ugly Wolf." A scene follows in which the Wolf goes to Grandma's house but Little Red Riding Hood finds him out, calls the Huntsman for help and together they chase him away. The grandmother, also impersonated by the therapist, compliments Little Riding Hood: "You are such a brave little girl, you were afraid but you knew how to be strong and defend yourself." Back home, Little Red Riding Hood faces further attacks from the Wolf and the Wicked Witch, directed against King Dad and Mummy Queen, calling a friend to assist her, but fighting in the first person; in the end, she manages to defeat the villains who run away. King Dad, in the voice of the therapist, says that Little Red Riding Hood was so afraid of losing Daddy and Mummy and finding the Wolf and the Wicked Witch in their place, but she did very well fighting and overcoming her fear. Now the Wolf has been driven away but, if he comes back, Little Red Riding Hood will know what to do. The session time is over, and on leaving, Emma says: "It feels good to play with you."

In the session, apart from an initial hello and Emma's final comment, there are only the words of the play, but between the child and the therapist all the indispensable contents have passed equally, and with great effectiveness, without the need to translate them into direct interpretive language: why Emma is there, what is her fear (losing her good parents replaced by persecutory bad figures). the request for help, the relief given by the hope of no longer being afraid.

Using touch

Just as words can "touch" through an embodied language that conveys emotions (Quinodoz, 2004). so too do gestures, touching the patient deep inside and conveying feelings that circulate in the relationship. Gestures in therapy are there, some are (apparently) simple and habitual, like the handshake during greetings, others unusual like the embrace, and all of them put in direct communication the world of the therapist's affections with that of the patient. They often, but not always, arise spontaneously, and it is still up to the therapist to understand with whom, and if and when they are necessary and appropriate, what their meanings and effects are on the relationship and the working process.

The habitual handshake on arriving or leaving attests to the desire to see each other and work together, it sanctions the therapeutic alliance, with mutual acceptance; some patients may need it to feel encouraged or feel that the therapist is not too cold and distant; for others, however, the same gesture represents an inappropriate invasion, and so the therapist, even if accustomed to greeting patients in this way, must understand it and abstain. Even small everyday gestures or actions may be inappropriate for certain patients or for the moment the therapeutic couple is going through; in such cases, they cause small cracks in the relationship, ruptures in the alliance, sometimes even pathological collusions (McWilliams, 2004). It is up to the psychotherapist to heal these cracks, to be aware of them, to understand the outcomes, to adjust the course of one's actions.

In the following case we see that it is precisely the therapist's awareness of having made an inappropriate gesture and her sincerity in talking to the patient about it that open up a new and more authentic path for therapy.

Elena: the unwelcome touch

One therapist, used to shaking hands when entering the room, sensing the reluctance of Elena,[7] a very defensive patient, had stopped doing so with her. Once, however, without consciously thinking about it, she offered her hand to the patient, who, although reluctant, returned it. The therapist then apologised to her, expressing her perception that she had disturbed her with unwelcome physical contact. The therapist had been immediately aware of her own "acting in", probably dictated by a desire for more communication and closeness with the patient, and she made use of her awareness, through her apology, to open an area of truthfulness, which proved to be a harbinger of new explorations.

Elena, in fact, first explicitly confirmed the unwelcome sensation and said, with a certain aggressiveness, that she did not like "being touched", but shortly afterwards she began to recount some phobic symptoms hitherto kept hidden, including the need to move to the couch to avoid the heat left by the previous patient, commenting on it with an expression of revulsion. The exploration of this repugnance led to a traumatic memory from early adolescence: her father aroused her disgust and disapproval since she had discovered pornographic material among his things and, interpreting every gesture or word of her father as an attempt at seduction, she prevented herself from approaching him. As an adult, her romantic relationships, interspersed with a few fleeting encounters of an exclusively sexual nature, were characterised by her partner's prevarication towards her, with some experiences of abuse and beatings. For her, physical proximity and bodily gestures or touching, were intrusive, persecutory, abusive.

Through her apology, the therapist was able to re-establish a respectful, protective distance for Elena, and tactfully gave recognition and voice to her fears.

In the course of therapy, there may be moments of particular pathos when words are superfluous or insufficient to convey all the emotional intensity; then it is only a gesture that is needed.

Paolo's parents: melting in the embrace

At the moment of saying goodbye at the end of an interview, when Paolo,[8] their child, who had been undergoing a long and difficult psychotherapy for some time, was finally overcoming the serious behaviour that had been troubling them so much, the weeping mother embraced the therapist and the father joined them, enclosing them with his arms. The therapist recounts:

> I did not think of shirking. In that moment, all the pains of those terrible years passed in front of us like a film and we experienced them together again, but then, as if washed away by the tears that finally flowed freely, we saw them fade away, giving way to relief and trust; I was united with them by my affection for the child and by the sharing of the pain, and they must have felt it.

Let us also think of the work with severely traumatised patients, who are in mourning, who fall seriously ill, or who suffer serious losses during therapy: sometimes lightly touching an arm, shaking a hand, responding to a hug, transmit that sympathy and solidarity that, even before belonging to the role of therapist, belong to him/her as a human being. After all, the encounter between a therapist and a patient is first and foremost an encounter between two persons even in the asymmetry of the relationship, and it is necessary that this humanity is always reciprocally kept in mind in order to provide relief from psychic pain, not only through therapeutic empathy and interpretative work, but also, at times, through direct and courageous moments of real sharing, explicitness and self-disclosure (Lapi, 2021).

Non-verbal language, if carefully observed in the patient and in oneself, and consciously used, becomes an effective tool of therapeutic dialogue, especially when the patient's words do not convey authenticity but are a curtain that hides and prevents one from thinking,[9] or when a massive and tenacious silence deprives the therapist of words.

Francesca: talking hands

F. Mori, in his (1993) pioneering work on silence, remembers himself, as a young analyst, in the therapy of a psychotic, mutacic girl: listening to his own emotional resonance led him to make use of non-verbal action, the only means of engaging in a communicative exchange with the patient:

> Francesca was brought to me when she was 24 years old, after having undergone all possible shock and psychopharmacological treatments ... The communications I had with her I can't say were poor, but they were certainly non-verbal and little articulated ... she would often spend the whole time standing, in silence, her back leaning against the entrance door ... sometimes an eye fixed on me, among the leaves of a plant ... I found myself resenting this presence so closed ... so blocked, myself, blocked, helpless, quivering ... I resolved to tell her, accompanying my words with action, that I felt I was not counteracting the desire I had to use my hands in order to try to open hers, to try to understand from her muscular reaction what reception she was making to what I was telling her ... her hands were allowing themselves to be opened by mine, and they did not escape contact. Palm against palm, fingers against fingers ... a quivering, a stiffening, a loosening, a wriggling, a closing, a retreating, which meant authentic reactions to me.
>
> (Mori, 1993)

This poignant and intense tactile language, with an authentically psychoanalytic value in that context, allowed Francesca not to hide and not to run away, and the analyst to feel alive; a dialogue opened up between them, made up of emotions that had finally found expressivity and that it was possible for the analyst to understand and give meaning to them; later words also arrived and the analysis went on, but first it took this time, the long time of action.

In psychotherapy, touch is used to communicate emotions, otherwise not transmissible with the same intensity, as in the case of Paolo's parents, and to know in depth when other means fail, as in the case of Francesca. Precisely from these clinical cases we note what is its particularity, unique with respect to the other senses: its being, so to speak, bidirectional. In fact, the moment one touches, one is touched, the particularities of the other are perceived and understood through our own perceptions, the body of the Other is perceived through our body. It is a circularity that becomes in itself a dialogue in which the two actors are at the same time subjects and objects, perceivers and receivers of perceptions: in the embrace and in the tears it is not possible to distinguish the perceptions of Paolo's parents from those of the therapist. When the analyst touches Francesca to get to know her and make her feel wanted, we sensed how moved he was by the tremors and flickers of her hands.

Touching, therefore, is a powerful medium that involves both the patient and the therapist in full "field" (Ferro, 1996). and precisely because it is so powerful, it can also become dangerous involvement, and therefore requires great restraint in its management. Not by chance, in its figurative sense, in the Italian language "touch" is synonymous with "tact", which indicates "shrewdness, gentleness in acting, the ability to behave with discretion and diplomacy" (*Enciclopedia Treccani*, 2021).

From Ferenczi, we learnt that behaving tactfully is useful in therapeutic work:

> Tact is the capacity for "empathy" … this empathy will prevent us from provoking the patient's resistance unnecessarily or at the wrong moment: even if psychoanalysis cannot completely spare suffering, one of its main achievements consists in teaching how to bear pain. On the contrary, if we are tactless and exert pressure on the patient without regard, we will offer him precisely that opportunity which in his unconscious he so ardently desires: that of evading our influence.
>
> (2002)

This therapeutic tact must also be used in the gestures of touching so as not to provoke feelings of intrusion, distancing, or collusion and misunderstanding that can make the therapist, the patient, and the process become ill.

Different words

There are words that do not belong to our psychoanalytic lexicon, nor to the familiar lexicon which is developed in the therapeutic relationship and connotes it with its specific idioms: they are "different" words, which at particular moments produce important events in the therapeutic process, with a pragmatic effect such as a gesture or an interpretative action would produce.

The obese adolescent

Words belonging to everyday life can suddenly arise from the spontaneity of a deep empathic resonance, as in the case of an obese adolescent treated by Pellizzari (2002). This is a young man with serious relational and behavioural difficulties, who fills all the sessions with a frenetic agitation of body and mind. The therapist is unable to stop the uninterrupted river of his words to get in intimate contact with him, until "suddenly he tells me that that very day was his birthday and that he had not invited anyone. Instinctively and with great warmth I say to him: 'Best wishes!'" These simple and spontaneous words have the effect of calming the boy, who remains silent for the first time, and then says, moved: "Fifteen years thrown away!" The words "best wishes" concretely reveal the therapist's affectionate closeness to the boy who, no longer feeling alone, can let his aching Self speak: "This allows him to get closer, because his persecutory fears have been disproved, and to begin to reflect on himself by facing painful awareness, but now made more tolerable by the presence of another who can understand him."

At other times, it is the therapist who consciously chooses the strategy of talking with the patient about literature, cinema, painting, music, and with adolescents about songs, sports, video games: drawing on other fields of their own experience, opens up a communicative channel, otherwise closed, creating a potential space of play where the patient and therapist can meet lightly, testing the ability to understand each other and experiencing contact without activating fear.

There are patients who find it very difficult to recognise and tolerate their feelings of transference, perhaps because they are particularly intense, and interpretations on this provoke rejection and closure. It is not uncommon, however, that the use of words belonging to fields other than psychoanalysis, apparently neutral but powerful vehicles of meanings in the interpsychic flow, activate a sharing between people that chases away fantasies of power and intrusion, and creates the basis for an alliance, that "we" that makes it possible to work together.

Antonio: finally, the "us"

Antonio,[10] a young man with a deficiency in primary relationships and a very rigid superego, goes through recurrent states of anxiety-depression, caught up in dutiful ideals of perfection, linked to a very rigid and judgmental maternal image, and the helpless feeling of always being wrong.

After more than a year of single-weekly sessions, he still maintains a critical detachment from psychotherapy, with continuous attacks on its effectiveness, and refusal of the offer to intensify the number of sessions. The most tenacious refusal is towards the emotions circulating in the relationship, especially when, together with anger and the fear of being invaded, a small dangerous hot current of curiosity and sympathy towards the therapist begins to leak out, which is, however, immediately afterwards rigidly denied. Woe, in fact, to speak of it: any mention of transference interpretations, however cautious, provokes in him reactions of closure and estrangement, arousing in the psychotherapist the image of the Mimosa Pudica, that sensitive plant that recoils at the touch. On the eve of a trip for a rather painful reason related to his family, which will keep him away from psychotherapy for a few sessions, Antonio suddenly asks the therapist for advice about a book to read during the long hours on the train; a short but unusually relaxed and lively conversation ensues, about the books he has recently read and both of their tastes in reading. At the end of the session, the therapist thinks of a book she had read many years before, when she was about the patient's age, which she had enjoyed very much, and without thinking too much about it, she tells the patient the title.[11]

On his return, at the end of the session, Antonio says he could not find the book. The therapist feels disappointed and wonders whether she should have refrained from acting in by recommending a book, moreover, one unobtainable by the patient: perhaps she had resistance to making a part of herself available to the patient? Perhaps she acted like a mother who does not let the child find her? And, again, perhaps the patient, not finding that book/part of her, made her feel as she always felt with her own mother: a child not found, not read/understood by an out-of-touch mother? A child trying to be perfect but always getting it wrong?

The therapy continues for a few more weeks, but even though Antonio finds it difficult to talk about the grief he experienced during the family visit and shifts his grief elsewhere, the climate of the relationship is remarkably relaxed, there is an emotional thaw.

Then, the Christmas break and, on his return, the surprise: a gift from Antonio, made by him during the holidays, accompanied by a card with hopeful words that admit his closure but also his desire. He comments, in fact: "I wrote it just thinking of us, a message-object to myself and to you to help me." The moving moment of saying "us" has arrived: something began to loosen up when the therapist gave something of herself by recommending the book, and now Antonio too was able to give something of himself, finally something related to the sphere of those feelings that frighten him and that he tries to keep tenaciously under control, but on which it will now be possible to start working together.

The child/patient and mother/therapist found each other.

Sharing, even the kind which takes place in the patient's and the therapist's real life, can be a necessary step in the therapeutic process to discover new and unknown areas or to overcome prolonged states of resistance, especially with those patients like Antonio, with primary deficiencies and disturbances in contact with themselves (Bolognini, 2002).

Talking outside the strictly therapeutic work of free associations and interpretations can have a profound transformative effect, even with patients with severe borderline and narcissistic personality structures, who lack the ability to dream[12] and to whom the therapist must in a certain sense lend his or her mind. To the extent that the therapist shares cultural interests with the patient, these common interests create a space of shared pleasure, an intermediate area that also helps the therapist to tolerate the patient's toxic projective identifications, to continue to feel alive and to transmit vitality to the patient and the relationship (Fano Cassese, 2010).

Taking care of the process

Two clinical narratives serve to illustrate how actions – the shared enactment of Jacobs and patient N., the language of gestures in Igor and Gaia's therapy – can heal the relationship and the process, resolving impasses and revitalising the therapy.

Jacobs and N.: caressing

After the emergence of an interesting content (the memory of having been subjected to abusive caresses by a cousin as a child). N., a very difficult young patient, for several sessions closes herself off in a defensive speech without content. In one particularly empty session, Jacobs, seized by deep boredom, picks up his pad and strokes its rib before taking notes, making a slight noise. N. notices this and complains about the analyst's distraction saying: "I felt like he was caressing something." Jacobs, the therapist, merely points out to her the use of the word "caressing" and N., in return, understanding Jacobs' association with the episode of her cousin, begins to talk about it, albeit in polemical and angry tones with Jacobs, confirming that she feels very disappointed in him; the analysis continues in its stalemate also in the following sessions. Then Jacobs, reflecting on the episode, realises that:

> Rather than shamefully acknowledging the accuracy of her perceptions and thus experiencing the associated feelings of guilt and shame, I had lured her down a different path. And for reasons of her own, which had much to do with her fear of a confrontation fraught with danger, she had followed me … in an unconscious enactment I had played the role of cousin in an attempt to stimulate the reappearance of the patient's communications.

However, as relevant as these objectives were, it was also true that both the patient and the analyst had resorted to them in order to avoid a confrontation that would generate – for both of them – much heavier states of anxiety. Jacobs understands that he must take up and clarify this episode with N. in order to regain her trust. He then tells her, explicitly, that her perception of his distraction was correct, and that he had been too embarrassed to admit it, but that it is now time to confront those hidden communications which had led Jacobs to feel boredom and N. to flee. The shared enactment for N. was to avoid feeling a strong anger towards her analyst, and the consequent fear that if she expressed it, Jacobs would become angry in turn and abandon her – as her love objects had abandoned her in the past; for Jacobs, it was to avoid a nasty narcissistic wound. Jacobs decided to expose himself, however, as "it would be a serious failing not to recognise an error, or to overlook the fact that a certain collusion had taken place between patient and analyst and that – because of this – the therapy had undergone a particular deviation".

The explanation of all this allowed the exploration of unconscious conflicts present in N. and Jacobs, hitherto concealed: "And it was this exploration, initiated and made possible by the unconscious communications, expressed as enactment, that allowed the therapy to advance towards healing, of the patient and the analyst" (Jacobs, 1986).

Igor and Gaia: the betrayal of words

Igor and Gaia[13] come from two different foreign countries and are in weekly psychotherapy for their marital crisis. The therapist's listening is difficult right from the start: she seems unable to understand and communicate adequately, especially with Igor, who shows open resistance to the treatment, and her countertransference experiences are of powerlessness, difficult emotional attunement, and the feeling of being constantly misunderstood. Igor, at one point, makes explicit the communication problem that weighs on the therapy, as the therapist recounts:

> Igor summarizes the issue of the different languages we use: Gaia speaks Ukrainian, as well as Italian, and also well; Igor speaks Moldovan but, in addition to Italian, also Ukrainian, because his maternal grandmother, a significant figure, was Ukrainian; I speak Italian, the language with which we communicate. "With Italian, you cannot say the things of the heart," says Igor. "Only with your native language, the mother tongue, can you really say the things you feel." Italian, he points out, forces them to move away from their emotions. We try to play with the various possible combinations of languages and translations to be used in the session, to conclude that it would not even be useful for him to speak in Ukrainian and for Gaia to translate into Italian for me since she would have to know all the words in Italian (he now uses the word "tradire"– which means to betray, instead of "tradurre"[14]). I then assume that, as for me, it is quite clear to Igor and Gaia that we should not rely too much on words, in any language, since "we would only end up betraying one another anyway". Igor proposes that we try, then, to rely on each other, as in a game, perhaps ... on the language of gestures: the finger firmly planted in the middle of the cheek marked by the scar, will then mean that "something is good", while the hand that swings nearer and farther away from the chest, with the fingertips pointing upwards and clasped together, will mean, in a hasty way, "what do you want?". With the gesture of children who do not yet know how to speak, I say that they are signalling to me the importance of being able to communicate to each other in the meantime what they may like and what they each wish to receive. Igor will remember the first word in Italian that their child learnt: "mama". Gaia, on the other hand, will remember the first words she heard their little girl say: "mi dai" (give me). They laugh amusedly.
>
> (Iorio, 2020)

Here we see how resorting to action, abandoning verbal language for a moment to use body language, managed to reach primary levels of experience, resolving the impasse in psychotherapy. The therapist, actively participating in this game of recovering the preverbal and universal mother-tongue, accepted to use with them a communicative level equivalent to the first mother-child relationships, which skips the conscious and interpersonal ego to become interpsychic. The recovery of the use of the primary language, the only one with which one can say the "words of the heart", was the experience divided between the therapist and the couple, which allowed Igor and Gaia to open up to the recovery of traumatic memories and unprocessed grief belonging to their youth and their families of origin, with, at last, full trust in the therapist's listening and containment.

Psychotherapy as "doing together"

> During a session in which I again found the child withdrawn and reluctant to respond, I left her, telling her I would be right back. I went to my children's room and took some toys, cars, figurines, bricks and a toy train, put them in a box and returned to the patient. The child, who had not yet begun to draw or do anything else, became interested in the toys and immediately started to play.
>
> (Klein, 1953 [1986])

Child psychoanalysis began that day, and it began with an action.

Children's therapy has always been a different kind of therapy, which has never been conditioned by the much-demonised acting-out, or the "white screen": the therapist involves himself with the child with his whole self, body and mind, playing with him on the carpet, bathing at the sink, accompanying him to the bathroom and using if necessary those "special technical methods" recommended by Klein even then, to overcome, for example, inhibitions or acute crises: "and she started screaming, showing all the symptoms of a severe crisis of anxiety. So, I sat down at the toy table and began to play by myself, describing to the child what I was doing" (Klein, 1953 [1986]).

Thinking back to these beginnings, which are still so topical, can help us to use the spontaneity of therapeutic feeling and empathic movements without fear and prejudice, drawing useful lessons from our work with children and adolescents to ensure that ours is a psychotherapy that heals (also) with actions.

Clara: untying the knots

One example is Clara's therapy, narrated in the first person by the therapist.

Clara[15] is a 10-year-old girl whom I follow in weekly therapy; from the very first meeting I felt a deep anxiety, a sense of desperation and loneliness, I am struck and saddened by her neglect (an expression of the difficulties in her relationship with her mother) and her silence, which will last for years, in which I feel lost, sometimes blocked, and can only communicate with her with drawings or small written phrases.

The entire course of therapy was marked by gestures, right from the first session: it was Clara who chose me by giving me, on the door, before she left, a paper doll with the words: "I Love You".

Clara has great difficulty in asserting herself, because she perceives this as a destructive gesture towards her mother, and in therapy it therefore emerges in hidden ways, in the drawings we make together, or in the sentences written on pads that I make for her so that she can deposit the various expressions of herself in them without being too frightened by them.

Our therapy – and I say "our" because we built it together, letting myself be guided by the patient, trying to listen to her with all my senses and devoting a lot of time, a lot of thought, to our work, both before and after the sessions – is a "doing together" therapy. Clara for a time used the space of the sessions to do her homework, I would learn new things together with her (her school performance improved considerably) and she would say: "Doing homework with you does me a lot of good!"

Another game she repeatedly asked me to play was doing experiments: Clara was the scientist trying to discover how the world around her works (an excellent metaphor for therapy): "It's nice to come here! In this silence, thoughts are released!", testifying to the experience she can finally have of herself, no longer a prisoner of fear.

It is within this context that the episode I am going to describe fits: after about three years of therapy, during a session, I perform a gesture, an action, which leaves me dismayed, but which I perceive as essential to communicate with the patient.

Clara arrives with her head down, she is silent and does not look at me; she rests her arms on the desk as if to support herself, she does not propose anything (it is usually she who introduces the theme-action of the meetings). I remark aloud that there seems to be something weighing on her; I ask her if she feels sad, she nods, but does not look at me or speak. It has been a long time since I saw Clara like this: a prisoner of her silence, seemingly eager to disappear into herself. I ask her if something has happened at home, with her parents, if she has had a fight with her mother (which sometimes happens, but of which I am usually promptly warned). Slowly I try to understand what is happening to her. She confirms to me that she is feeling down but is rather tenacious in avoiding contact with me. At one point she unties her hair (she had it in a ponytail) and shows me a knotted lock: "That's why," she says, "I didn't want you to see it because you'll think I'm a lousy person who doesn't wash." I look at her, taking the huge tangle of hair in my hands. It seems to me an arduous task to untangle it, but also urgent, necessary. It seems to me that all that tangle well represents the patient's emotional states, the thoughts that cluster together creating a tight tangle that prevents them from being encoded, and which imprisons her and reduces her to a condition of miserable helplessness. I could tell her all these things, but would it help? How to transform the patient's knots/thoughts? As these thoughts run through my mind, one thread after another I try to retrace the movements of the hair backwards and attempt, slowly, to untie them. I am reminded of the legend of Medusa, transformed into a monster by Athena because she had dared to compete with her in beauty (I think of Clara's relationship with her own mother and what she is doing with me in the transference). I make a comment on the quality of her hair, and I verbalise, staging a kind of theatre, what I am doing, asking her for help because she is the one who knows her hair and can help me understand it. We search together for the meaning of that big knot. While this is going on, Clara can finally talk about another "knot", the one stemming from her relationship with her mother, which generates whirlpools of anger in which she remains imprisoned: "Mum is unpredictable, when I ask her something I never know what she's going to answer, it can be that it's OK and she answers me in a nice way, or she tells me 'No!' in a rude way, without explaining why ... All this confuses me and makes me angry." Together we reconstruct the two reactions that she has when she feels anger towards her mother: the depressive one (closure) when she is denied something and feels miserable and undeserving (deprived and unable to arouse thoughtfulness in others), and the uncontrolled anger (which does not make her think and makes her want to kill herself) when she feels judged and criticised by her mother.

In the sessions following this one, Clara will be able to talk about her needs and the suffering she has experienced due to the dissatisfaction of these needs (the disappointed need for a warm and caring family). the many emotions that run through her (she will make a drawing that she will call "Strange Life" and will tell me that it represents herself thinking about many emotions) and the urge to try and invest in herself (she becomes passionate about studying and starts wearing make-up).

Through the action of untying, Clara was able to experience a transformative dimension that allowed her to express in words her "tangled" experiences (experiences that can be thought of as also present in the transference). Untangling the knot was an attempt to free her from her anger and legitimise its constructive aspects, handing her a method with which she could try to retrace her own experiences by untangling the conflictual knots (once the knot was untangled, she could go on by herself in taking care of her own hair/thoughts).

We see realised in child psychotherapy, in Clara's and all our young patients' treatments, that this "doing-together psychotherapy" where thoughts are released in the silence of words (to use the child's expression) and symbolic meanings do not necessarily need verbal representation to be communicated. Symbolisation is expressed by the body and its sensory transmissions, by actions, by play, in which the therapist actively participates, co-actor of the action, and from session to session it is the child-therapist couple that puts together and co-constructs the story.

If this is the natural way of expressing oneself with children, other subjects, as we have said, can benefit from this way of psychotherapy: subjects with serious symbolic defects, narcissistic pathologies, pathologies that undermine identity, affected by early trauma, producing body-expressed or acted-out symptoms.

Sailing to distant lands

> Interpretive action is not an exceptional analytical event, it is simply part of the fabric of ordinary interpretive analytical work.
>
> (Ogden, 1994)

We know that therapeutic work is continually studded with difficult moments: impasses, enactments, blind areas whose aim is to shelter both patient and therapist from intolerable anxieties but which also create ramparts that stand in the way of growth (Ferro, 1996). We have learnt, however, that it is possible to use these facts to turn them in favour of new developments by recognising and interpreting them, and now we are already on to the next step: that of considering them as therapeutic tools.

The way of considering the therapist's actions in the session – from a dangerous mistake to a therapeutic tool, as Ogden (1994) teaches us – well represents the different way of thinking that is taking place in psychoanalysis and psychotherapy, which overturns our usual perspective and teaches us not to be afraid.

Inevitably present in the relationship, actions must be admitted if, acknowledged, used without too much fear of contacting the patient so directly and intimately. Relying on actions is undoubtedly difficult and risky: when is it an action that cures and when is it an acting-in that makes one ill? There is a narrow line between them, and almost always, unfortunately, only traceable in retrospect. The risk, which has always been feared, is still the same: colluding with the pathology and affecting the field. Unmanaged emotions can cause us to slide off the analytical terrain towards a factual reality where it is possible to act but not to listen and contain: indeed, "When too much reality and too much action enter therapy, suddenly listening stops" (Goisis, 2020). Losing the therapeutic frame of mind in the action may lead us to the risk of violating, more or less unconsciously, the boundaries, certainly of the setting and technique and, in extreme cases, even those of our code of ethics. The therapist must manage to be so good as to allow himself to be involved but at the same time preserve his "second glance" (Baranger et al., 1993; Ferro, 1996): that ability to observe the therapeutic field while being part of it, placing himself in a sort of supervision of himself and carrying out a very close monitoring of the patient's responses and of the relationship's strength.

The temptation in the face of such complexity might be to turn back and take defensive refuge in the exclusivity of interpretation. The "Scylla and Charybdis" between which the therapist must wisely navigate, are ultimately the same as those between which psychoanalytic therapists have always navigated: valorising non-interpretive therapeutic factors or considering interpretation as the sole, authentic, effective therapeutic instrument. The current clinical experience of psychoanalytic psychotherapies warns us against idealising interpretation, which leads to not giving due value to all the other, albeit effective, tools available to the therapist, and which, moreover, can also be used for defensive and distancing purposes, to the detriment of the treatment relationship.

We still have much to study and research, without pretending to arrive immediately at definitions that, instead of bringing certainty, would produce rigidity; rather, we must remain open to new mental constructions by tolerating uncertainty, exercising negative capacity, relying from time to time on the course that guides that specific relationship with that specific patient.

Carried by the wind of the desire for knowledge, and not by that of emotional gratification, the course will be safer and, having overcome "Scylla and Charybdis", navigation can continue with the aid of new instruments such as action, alongside, of course, the classic ones. Sometimes it will be a consciously meditated action, most often it will spring spontaneously from our therapeutic responsiveness in those precious moments of interpsychic communication that occasionally occur in good psychotherapy.

With gestures that touch and actions that heal, we can then reach those areas of the patient that are deaf to our words, like distant lands hitherto unreachable by our voice.

Notes

1 See also the IPA's *Inter-regional Encyclopaedic Dictionary of Psychoanalysis* (IPA, 2021), available at: www.ipa.world/IPA/IPA_Docs/PDFDocuments/SET TING-Italian%20final%20edited.pdf; Panizza's (2013) text; the numerous works by Baranger *et al.* (1993) and A. Ferro (1996). These themes were also the focus of several papers at the 19th SPI Congress, "Unconscious. Unconscious", 4–7 February 2021, Rome.
2 As we shall see later, in T. Jacobs' interesting clinical exemplification of an enactment of analyst and patient leading to a positive turn in analysis.
3 These issues are particularly addressed in Chapters 2 and 6.
4 It is thus, for example, that a patient with a "psychic skin" defect is given the prescription to wear in her moments of greatest distress a woollen poncho (chosen by her but given to her by her parents) that can wrap and contain her as a second skin (Racamier, 1997).
5 The case was treated by A. Corotti, a student at the AFPP School, whom we thank for providing the clinical material.
6 The case was treated by I. Lapi.
7 The case was treated by S. Pampaloni.
8 The case was treated by I. Lapi; for the case description, see Chapter 2.
9 We refer to those patients who flood the sessions with fluent but empty speech, as in the case described below of an obese adolescent.
10 The case was treated by I. Lapi.

11 As was to be expected, the title chosen was very much related both to Antonio's psychic situation and to the therapist's personal affairs … a co-constructed choice of field.
12 See Chapter 6.
13 The case was treated by I. Iorio (2020).
14 Igor's slip actually recalls a certain view of translation ("tradurre") as a betrayal ("tradire") of the original word when transforming it into something else (Amrhein, 2012).
15 The case was treated by E. Di Mauro.

References

Amrhein, J. (2012). Questions à Freud sur la traversée de l'abîme. *Insistance*, 7: 43–53.
Baranger, M., Baranger, W. and Mom, J.M. (1993). Processo e non processo nel lavoro analitico. *Ricerca Psicoanalitica*, VIII(1): 97–118.
Bolognini, S. (2002). *L'empatia psicoanalitica*. Turin: Bollati Boringhieri.
Bolognini, S. (2008). *Passaggi segreti*. Turin: Bollati Boringhieri.
Bolognini, S. (2019). *Flussi vitali tra Sé e Non-Sé. L'interpsichico*. Milan: Raffaello Cortina.
Enciclopedie Treccani (2021). Available at: https://www.treccani.it/enciclopedia/elen co-opere/Enciclopedie_on_line/ (accessed 10 May 2021).
Etchegoyen, R.H. (1986). *Los fundamentos de la técnica psicoanalitica*. Buenos Aires: Amorrortu Editores.
Fano Cassese, S. (2010). L'interpretazione ispirata e parlare come sognare. Available at: www.spi-firenze.it/l-interpretazione-ispirata-e-parlare-come-sognare-silvia-fano-cassese/ (accessed 6 November 2020).
Ferenczi, S. (2002). L'elasticità della tecnica psicoanalitica. In S. Ferenczi, *Opere*, vol. IV. *1927–1933*. Milan: Raffaello Cortina.
Ferro, A. (1996). *Nella stanza d'analisi*. Milan: Raffaello Cortina.
Freud, S. (1938 [2001]). Introduction to Psychoanalysis. In J. Strachey (ed.), *The Complete Psychological Works of Sigmund Freud*, vol. XXIII*(1937–1939)*. London: Hogarth Press.
Goisis, P.R. (2020). *Nella stanza dei sogni*. Brescia: Enrico Damiani Editore.
Guerrini Degli Innocenti, B. (2017). Parole in azione. Available at: www.spi-firenze.it (accessed 4 April 2021).
Iorio, I. (2020). L'ascolto transgenerazionale della coppia. In Soci Italiani EFPP, *L'ascolto psicoanalitico. Efficacia e fattori terapeutici della psicoterapia*. Rome: Alpes.
IPA (2021). *Inter-Regional Encyclopedic Dictionary of Psychoanalysis*. Available at: www.ipa.world (accessed 3 May 2021).
Jacobs, T.J. (1986). On trasferente enactments. *Gli Argonauti*, 33: 89–103.
Jacobs, T.J. (2001). Delphinium blu e gerani rossi. *Gli Argonauti*, 88: 3–26.
Klein, M. (1953 [1986]). La tecnica psicoanalitica del gioco: sua storia e suo significato. In F. Fornari (ed.), *Fantasmi, gioco, società*. Milan: Il Saggiatore.
Lapi, I. (2021). Tematiche del dolore. *Contrappunto*, 60/61: 18–30.
McWilliams, N. (2004). *Psychoanalytic Psychotherapy: A Practitioner's Guide*. New York: Guilford Publications.
Mori, F. (1993). Quando difetta il linguaggio verbale nella coppia paziente-terapeuta. *Contrappunto*, 59: 12–32.

Nicolò, A.M. (2019). Al di là dell'interpretazione. Note sul cambiamento della tecnica in psicoanalisi. Available at: www.spi-firenze.it (accessed 25 February 2021).

Ogden, T.H. (1994). *Subjects of Analysis*. London: Routledge.

Panizza, S. (2013). *La prospettiva relazionale*. Milan: FrancoAngeli.

Pellizzari, G. (2002). *L'apprendista psicoterapeuta*. Turin:Bollati Boringhieri.

Prat, R. (2009). La preistoria della vita psichica: evoluzione e tracce nell'incontro e nel processo terapeutico. *Contrappunto*, 42: 75–94.

Prat, R. and Israel, P. (2013). Tra espressione verbale e espressione corporea: un approccio al trattamento psicoanalitico degli stati limite. *Contrappunto*, 48: 27–40.

Quinodoz ,D. (2004). *Les mots qui touchent*. Paris: Presses Universitaires de France.

Racamier, J.P. (1997). Una comunità di cura psicoterapeutica. Riflessioni a partire da un'esperienza di vent'anni. In A. Ferruta, G. Foresti, M. Vigorelli and E. Pedriali (eds), *La comunità terapeutica. Tramito e realtà*. Milan: Raffaello Cortina.

Winnicott, D.W. (1971). *Playing and Reality*. London: Tavistock Publications.

Chapter 5

New territories for the patient

The therapist's dreams

Stefania Pampaloni

Introduction

The choice to explore these themes represents my point of view on the Table of Thoughts, my curiosity and the questions I drew from it. Each of us followed a track from among those that emerged during the group work, mine was a reflection on the therapist's authenticity, of which I seem to succinctly grasp both the intersubjective aspects and the reflection on the body; the authenticity of the therapist who participates as a subject, with a variety of self-expressions, already considered as peculiar characteristics of the psychoanalytic therapist. This starting point is connected to a search that is directed towards the therapist's own internal world, to the point of encountering possible obstacles to one's therapeutic functions.

The encounter with the patient's unprocessed, traumatic areas, relegated to the body, call the therapist's mind back to his own representations, sufficiently or insufficiently worked out and it is precisely those areas that dialogue with deep aspects of the therapist, from unconscious to unconscious. It is an encounter that revives one's own pathways, and that can raise defences or suffering, and if not recognised and worked through, risks weakening the primary functions of the therapeutic relationship: containment and dreaming (together).

The function of containment recalls and re-processes the first experiences of caregiving in the patient's life; this is a moment in the child's development that neuropsychological research is providing with new knowledge, illuminating also the concepts of introjection and installation in the body. Therefore, new attention is given to the body, not only of the patient but also of the therapist, to his actions and his subjectivity: it is the therapist's Self, with his body, his dreams and his personal history, that enters into the clinic, into theory and technique, into training and supervision.

The therapist's dream concerning the patient contains aspects of countertransference (dream countertransference), responsive to the transference implemented by the patient, but also elements of the therapist's own

DOI: 10.4324/9781032673721-6

subjectivity, of his personal history, which through listening and relating are recalled, an unconsciously shared scenario in which therapeutic working through takes place.

The idea running through this work is that the therapist's dream is fuelled by early traumatic aspects of the patient. The hypothesis is that early trauma makes the traumatic cores, intertwined with the domain of the body and not removed, even more inaccessible, and that they can only be contacted through the body, or through the dream, not only of the patient but also of the therapist.

Dreaming together within a safe container can allow the patient to represent other scenarios and see new territories. An amplification that also uses the tools of literary and representational art, myth, philosophy. The progress of psychoanalytic psychotherapy thus also requires comparison with disciplines close to psychoanalysis, and with cultures that are unfortunately still too distant, such as the oriental ones.[1]

The therapist's authenticity and the trauma of non-affection

The image underlying the reflection is that of the psychoanalyst focused on the meanings of the patient's narrative (interpretive side) and in which the orthodoxy of the setting may leave no room for the need for people contact, the therapeutic factors inherent in the relationship, such as containment and, in general, the personal characteristics of the therapist.

The therapist's authentic being allows the opening, the amplification of the gaze on the body, on action, on dreams. Authenticity, for a psychotherapist, can mean staying in touch with one's countertransference in the session and revisiting it after the session (*après coup*). which is expressed in bodily sensations and actions, countertransference dreams, thoughts and interpretations. In this way, the deepening of the therapist's meaning of authenticity connects different realms.

It was Ferenczi, who, in *Confusion of Tongues* (1982), placed the issue of the therapist's authenticity in a groundbreaking way at the basis of his position, which marked a theoretical and technical autonomy with respect to classical psychoanalysis. Ferenczi's concern was not to repeat the model of coldness and detachment that caused the trauma: it was to cure the patient.

The concept of trauma requires a definition precisely because it is widely used and in fact lies at the heart of the transition from the unpleasant event to the possibility of mental processing. Trauma originated from affective deficiency or deprivation, occurring at the origins of life, at a time when communication with the outside world through the body is strong, or even the only way of communicating.

The deprivation of contact with the other concerns both the bodily aspects, being embraced, looked at, fed, and the related omnipotent illusion, the magical illusion that protects the child from the premature awareness of its separateness from the mother, an amplification of self and of its own creativity, which the child experiences through attunement with its mother, and which needs to be gradually abandoned; otherwise a dissociation will be set in motion that will affect the body, the thought-body that precedes the possibility of a true thought about itself.

Ferenczi also laid the foundations for psychosomatics in this way, with *Thalassa*, considered by Balint to be an indispensable text for the study of this science.

Winnicott then amplifies Ferenczi's emphasis on affective relations and makes them a constitutive part of the "psychic skin", of the "me-not-me" boundary: "when all goes well, the skin becomes the boundary between the me and the not-me, the psyche has come to live in the soma".[2] The body divides and connects the internal world from the external world. Thus, the therapist explores himself in accepting the patient's drama and, without re-presenting the original trauma of the exclusion and rejection, he himself amplifies his own territories, also encountering his own traumas.

At the origin is the body

At the origin is the body, the mental processes are at the service of the body's needs, as Freud (1938 [2001]) had already discovered with drive theory, the bodily demands made on psychic life, needs that move towards fulfilment and drive to action; the body is the first to enter into the complex game of the intersubjective relationship with the adult who cares for the child in its long neoteny.

Neuroscience is bridging that "mysterious leap from the mind to the body" Freud spoke of in his "Introduction to Psychoanalysis" (1915–1917 [2002]). which at the time lacked the scientific tools necessary to be investigated.

Not only the body, there is also communication between unconscious at the beginning. Anna Ferruta (2011) reminds us, in this regard, of Fachinelli's extraordinary description of "direct non-verbal communication between unconsciouses experienced in the early stages of development and repeated in analysis". Today, neuropsychology also maintains that the relationship passes from the mother's right hemisphere (the basis of affective communication) to the child's forming right hemisphere.[3] Clara Mucci states:

> if a mother has traumatisation and bereavement that she has not resolved at the time she is engaged in caring for her child, the child takes in the mother's dissociated areas, as if there had been mistreatment, in a kind of traumatic graft ... The care goes through the neurobiological correlates produced by the brain from the gaze, the touch, the voice. Life is always interaction.
>
> (2020)

This has implications for technique. Mucci speaks of *embodied testimony*, which means using in therapy all parts of one's bodily and mental self in a journey from the body to the mind, from the right hemisphere to the left hemisphere, and then back to the affective right side, in a continuous integrated process. And even more suggestive is the theoretical path that Vincenzo Bonaminio (2017) traces from Freud to Bollas, on the unconscious communication between analysand and analyst.

From trauma to splitting

In the beginning there is also the omnipotence of thought that requires a gradual time for unravelling. Trauma lies along a continuum from lack or deprivation of primary care to maltreatment "by human hands" and, in order to be understood, must also take into account the omnipotent-magic thinking phase the child is in. The combination of the elements in the field can lead the child to experience emptiness, nameless dread. In other words, the traumas experienced have different intensities and effects (on the body and/or on thought) and depend simultaneously on the age of onset of the trauma (on which depends the amount of omnipotence put to one's own protection, which decreases over time) and on the type of trauma (trauma due to deprivation or lack of primary care, trauma by human hands, collective trauma). The *enveloppe* of omnipotence must be gradually abandoned; early rupture leaves the child unprotected against terror.

There are many attempts to give a name to that primordial state of all-encompassing fear that remains somewhere inside us, starting with the trauma of birth.[4] Not only naming it, but also describing its effects. To describe the effects of trauma, Freud speaks of splitting (1938 [2001]). while Ferenczi (1958) sees it more as death; Ferenczi says that the child ends up no longer believing in his or her bodily experience, "the whole sector of that experience disintegrates into a mass of atomised debris".

Survivors of abuse become the aggressors of their own body because in that body there is also identification with the abuser figure, and the body plays the role of the victim in that identification, a kind of other. The emotions connected to these positions of victim and persecutor together are feelings of depression, inferiority, shame, despair and self-loathing connected to the victim side, and anger, revenge, hatred and fury connected to the persecutor side. Ferenczi, as we said, emphasises that traumatisation is followed by the incorporation of the aggressor's aggression.

An illuminating example of an installation of traumatic content in the body is the dream of an adolescent patient who was sexually abused in childhood and presents with an algic disorder: "I felt something pressing in my chest, it was a foetus making space between the organs, pushing, and playing dangerously with my heart." Such experiences can result in psychosomatic illnesses and hypochondria.

Clinical example: F.

To illustrate such splitting and incorporation I will present a short clinical case.

The stuttering of F., a 29-year-old patient, introduces us to the theme of the split between emotions and their verbal representation, a disconnection between the physiological level (non-symbolic) and the cognitive-experiential level (symbolic). between a more archaic way of functioning of thought and a more articulate mode, mediated by language.

The first year of therapy with F. is dominated by a massive use of projection of the patient's internal conflicting feelings that leaves no room for observation of the internal world and for a deeper elaboration of the Self, a wall that seems insurmountable and that at times makes one lose hope. A constant element is the inability to care and love, to welcome and understand, which could reproduce the experience he had with his mother, who did not allow him freedom to express himself, through criticism, devaluation, taboos on any subject with libidinal content (sexuality, politics, play and entertainment). a relationship permeated by maternal depression. Emotional and relational distance where one expects acceptance, understanding of needs, encouragement, rêverie, loving help for growth. A disturbing representation. As is the memory of the father, intent on suppressing the cat born without a tail, and therefore "defective".

In the patient, the mental effort to maintain the split with these parts is costly, in terms of hyper-control, obsessive rituals, loss of cohesion and sense of self. When the patient's obsessive defences gave way, a first elaboration of unconscious contents related to aggression was possible. I presented F.'s case to the Balint Group[5] of the Istituto di Formazione Psicosomatica in Florence and, during the subsequent guided self-distancing experience, I came into contact with the patient's discomfort and fear of unconscious aggression through some "awakenings" accompanied by a physical sensation of fear similar to a "stomach clench", the same that the patient had described in one of the previous sessions. We listen not only to the expression of verbal meanings, but also to other levels of psychic expression, we listen "with all our senses" (Bastianini et al., 2021). The experience during the group, and the subsequent contact with the body, allowed me to experience, also through it, the feeling of fear that I had not yet been able to name with the patient: the fear of aggression and death.

The work with the therapist's body is fundamental to the therapy, the mind-body integration that the therapist manages to achieve functions as a catalyst for a possible integration of the patient, his way of being in the body is constantly perceived, seen and felt by the patient.

Remembering that the child's thought can be born thanks to another thought that contains it and stimulates it to produce links between sensory and thought elements, in the absence of such containment, thought atomises and in place of the empty spaces left by unconstituted or interrupted links, dead, split parts are incorporated (Ferenczi, 1958), as in stuttering, where silences interrupt the melody of the patient's speech, mute parts as a symbol of death.

The body is a vehicle of meaning and communication, even more so for patients who have had early traumatic experiences. The first experiences of care and containment (containing with the arms, with the voice, with the eyes and with thought itself) leave sensory, physical traces that can be metabolised and transformed into psychic content; or, if a proto-organisation of the child's self has not yet been achieved, in a pre-verbal phase, or contiguous-autistic as Ogden puts it,[6] and containment is inadequate, the mental metabolism cannot process the unpleasant physical experiences/information, particularly when these take on an extreme form, we arrive at what Winnicott calls *fear of breakdown*. The unprocessed unpleasant experiences, which the child tries to get rid of in the ways available to him, remain in the area of physical contents. In other words, the consequences of relational deprivation (of trauma) in the early stages of development, when there is no capacity to represent something or someone in its absence, generate bodily experiences that are not fulfilled, in which pain cannot be contained by the thought that can provide meaning and reassurance (e.g., thinking: it will soon pass), and produce a fragmentation, making it difficult to construct a plot in which to weave free associations and dreams that express meaning for the patient's internal world.

The case described is connected to the temporality of the trauma, to the fact that a traumatic event occurs at a time when the child has no possibility of coping with sorrow, or despair, with language and thought, and this takes us to the context of the primitive mind and the unrepressed unconscious. The patient, in fact, taking into account the maternal depression and paternal intransigence, the traits of emotional detachment and devaluation that characterised their relationship with their child, may have encountered a rejecting and traumatising environment from birth.

The repressed unconscious speaks to us through symbols that have been repressed but were previously somehow contained and, before being pushed into less accessible areas of the mind, were processed, albeit in a primordial way, at a first level of thinkability. The repressed unconscious, in fact, requires a quota of thought that allows for repression. Between alpha and beta there are levels of transformation, what exists before beta, bodily and sensory, beyond the primal limit of experience, will constitute the non-repressed unconscious. It may be precisely this, due to its intrinsic difficulty of symbolic translation, that dialogues on a bodily and dream level.

The therapist's dreams

The therapist's dreams, as well as enactments, the importance of the therapist's body and actions have received little attention until recently; today, however, they are receiving increasing attention:

today we go so far as to explore pre-subjective states of the Self ... and we are deeply interested in the concept of enactment, which many have recognised as the fourth royal road to the unconscious, after the dream, transference and countertransference.

(Bolognini, 2021)

Body, sleep dreams, waking dreams and interpretations represent a continuum from the absence of symbolic contents to their maximum use in the interpretative intervention. Dreams are situated in an intermediate zone that listens to the signals of the body (actual body and experienced body[7]) and transforms them into representation, with a greater contact with the unconscious – ours and the patient's – even when it comes to waking dreams. This chapter originally had the title "Countertransference dreams", but as I looked into how Paula Heimann, Donald Winnicott, Heinrich Racker, and others after them, broadened the concept, it seemed to me that the prefix "counter", placed the therapist in a defensive position that shielded him from working with his own subjectivity and authenticity. In the course of the years, countertransference has come to take on globalist connotations, including the subtle interweaving of reciprocal influences between patient and therapist concerning their subjectivity, which we can hardly study and identify (something which Ferenczi tried to do with his experimental mutual analysis). It is even more difficult because of the therapist's secrecy about their dreams about the patient, harbingers of unconscious meanings that cannot be controlled.

In 1965, Giovanni Hautmann described his own dream of a patient (in "Un esempio di controidentificazione proiettiva", presented at the Italian Psychoanalytic Society in 1965). which he considered to be the first reported in the SPI journal, a sign of the presence of the analyst's person, even in theoretical elaboration.

For an orientation in the more recent panorama, Section IV of *Il Pensiero Psicoanalitico Italiano* (Borgogno et al., 2017) traces some lines of development that begin with the transition *from analyst to person* (Nissim Momigliano, 1984), pass through the need to include the countertransference in order to understand the patient, understanding countertransference dreams as an important part of the therapist-patient dynamics that helps in the understanding of the parallel dynamics activated in the patient's internal world (Bolognini, 2008), and conclude with the acknowledgement of the therapist's subjectivity and intersubjectivity.

The therapist's dream, together with his or her affections, is a door to participate in the unconscious/unconscious dialogue, to find meanings that will be useful to the patient and that will also be useful to the therapist. The mental functioning of the analyst open to what is not yet known, which also destabilises his mental set-up, and which opens up new horizons of thinkability and reorganisation of the subject's psychic structures (Ferruta, 2020).

Clinical example: L. and F.

I will briefly describe some clinical elements preceding my dream concerning two patients.

L., a 40-year-old patient undergoing weekly psychotherapy, recalls in two consecutive sessions, first, the film, *V for Vendetta* [8] ("V" is a vigilante, a rebel, with a disfigured face, perpetually covered by a smiling mask, in a dystopian, totalitarian and repressive world, *à la* Orwell) and subsequently his mother's rejection of his "animalistic" contents represented in a drawing, which she forced him to erase; a mother unavailable to him, between angry outbursts and crying fits, but also affectionate, with whom L. seems to have established a "bond of union", as in a work by Escher that the patient quotes in the session, in which two faces, of a man and a woman, are made up of a spiral ribbon flowing into each other, as if to represent, in its most destructive side, an intrusion into the body and its splitting.

L., in a different way from F., is aware of his anger and sadistic-aggressive impulses which feed the "fire of shame". These emotions make him feel "a despicable being", he controls his anger together with his spontaneous emotional impulses; at times, he looks at a point in front of him while I speak and I hear my voice becoming more and more distant, then he becomes alert again.

In this context I had the following dream:

> I am inside a sort of trapdoor, a small underground room with a porthole opening at the top, like that of a submarine, on which a ladder is resting; next to me is my sister, a professional rescuer. I look up, towards the round opening, where a man appears, approaching with a broom in his hand ... a moment later he is busy fiddling with a can of petrol. I wake up.

The man with the petrol can is a work of dream condensation, initially he is patient F., then he turns into L., two levels of repressed anger, from unconscious aggression to a more evolved and partially conscious level. F., with the broom in his hand, conveys sadistic-anal contents, as frequent are his references to evacuation and to retaining faeces; then the sadistic gaze lights up and, only from that detail do I recognise, in the final part of the dream, L. and his enjoyment in inflicting pain.

I wonder if I have identified with internal objects of the patient,[9] a part of him that is the victim of sadistic attacks.

I think of when F. felt this way, in life, perhaps already at birth, as the round opening above his head reminds me. In fact, I see him as a child inside that rather cramped space, who in the world outside finds annihilation, with no other option but to succumb or flee, just as the therapist escapes into awakening, with her alert, rational mind. He has escaped in the control that has become obsessive, carrying with him contents of death that have remained intact, as in a chest. I also think of L.'s overpowering impulse, and

the scene takes on the sense of a representation of the victim and the persecutor, aspects present in both patients, and where in F. the feeling of being
oppressed prevails, the victim of the situations he experiences, and in L. the
desire to subdue.

In these condensed images the question arises as to what is the contribution
that concerns the therapist and what concerns the patient. Among these
polysemic characters I examine the aspects most closely related to the "reassuring" area of countertransference or projective counter-identification.

The object that the patient places within is recognised and represented at an
unconscious level through the dream, the memory of which places this representation in front of a first stage of thinkability. This makes it possible to be used
as an object, unless the therapist's ability to dream is overwhelmed by the emotional content of the dream, generating an *interrupted dream* (Ogden, 2005). The
awakening from the therapist's dream as an avoidance of the patient's aggression
re-proposes the patient's avoidance of his own aggression, enacted with splits,
also represented by the interrupted expression of his stuttering words.

It is not easy to distinguish what belongs to the therapist[10] and what is
stimulated in him by the patient, since one includes the other.[11] It can be
represented by an internal resonance, recognising that part of oneself that has
experienced and relocated similar painful and/or dysfunctional contents that
the patient brings.

I feel the representation of the dream as extraneous, but such a content does
not belong to the patient alone, I would not have been able to dream it otherwise; an internal recognition of what is present in the patient's internal world, a
communication between unconscious minds, an intersubjective representation.[12]

In this interweaving of the foreign and the familiar, reminiscent of the
Freudian uncanny, Semi comes to my aid:

> I believe that self-analysis also serves a narcissistic reintegration that
> consists not only in recognising what is one's own and what has been
> sneaked in, so to speak, but in recognising that what comes from the
> other is our own and that, in this way, our own events, old and perhaps
> entrenched conflicts, residues of headaches that we thought we had over-
> come, are also expressed and taken up again.
>
> (2017)

Or, I would add, that they had been but which require new elaborations, for
the unconscious is in a continuous work of signification. Even more, for
Bollas (1987). we cannot discriminate between the therapist's processing of
the patient and his own "disseminations", but we can consider the dream-
space as a particular type of unconscious holding environment.

These are the new territories that appear on the horizon and that can be so
used or shared.[13] I believe that the tools the therapist possesses can provide
the courage and desire to explore. In therapy, the subject of discourse is the

patient's experience, and the therapist's experience can be used as a vehicle for understanding it.

As I continued to delve into the dream in different supervision contexts, these occasions painted my dream with new nuances, allowing me to understand its most painful themes. A different interpretation of the dream[14] foregrounds its obsessional-anal vertex, the claustrum (Meltzer, 1992) which imprisons and makes it difficult to use creativity, imagination and feelings to freely associate in the search for meaning. I struggle to acknowledge that this could be an element of contact with the patient, an aspect recognised in me and therefore representable. Representability and subsequent elaboration that express the meaning of the therapeutic function of the mind.

Awakening from the dream signals the difficulty of staying (together with the patient) in the traumatic area, when there is not even a place and a time to experience a scene, experience it. And the new territories the therapist is able to dream can be that place, which the patient can "use", make his own, or which the therapist can use to understand him.

For example, in a patient's dream: "an expanse of grey ice, evoking solitude as far as the eye can see, 'perfect' absence of sound, colour, life". A territory hitherto unknown to the patient, and therefore not possible to populate, and which only through the therapist's gaze was it possible to approach different, richer and more contiguous landscapes.

The dream as a ferry, an organising current of reality, a "conveyor belt" through strong oceanic currents that give rise to atmospheric phenomena and the life cycle, which connects us with lived–not lived experiences; it could represent a map that signals emerging configurations at a particular stage of therapy.

Clinical example: T.

Another clinical example where a heuristic dream of the therapist appears is that of patient T., a young adult always striving to defend his autonomy, whose readiness to respond left no room for uncertainty, creative doubt and imagination. His concealed and buried psychological dependence manifested itself in a pernicious and unrecognised addiction to both light drugs and the periodic need to tattoo himself. Being contradicted or defeated in games and sports gave rise to sudden and violent aggressive reactions. In this patient, the *enveloppe* of omnipotence had never been shaken in the first years of life, experienced by T. at the centre of the condescending attentions of parents, grandparents and aunts. After the description of him as a child inseparable from his blanket, we had shared the image of Linus, and it was the first time we had managed to portray a dependent, childlike aspect of him.

After the immersion, shared in the session, in the image of Linus I had the following short dream:

T. is sitting on a bench, a doctor friend of mine, retired a few months ago, who lost his elderly mother a few days ago, approaches him and sits down next to him.

This dream gave new clarity to the rejection of dependency (and the manifestation of counter-dependency) and at the same time signalled the deepening of the therapeutic relationship. It also gave substance to fleeting descriptions of the patient's relationship with his own mother, shedding light on hitherto unheard aspects of dependency, obscured by a resolute attitude, in the absence of empty spaces and silences in which unsolicited responses are immediate and certain.

Expansions to other languages

There remain, however, confused, blind areas, something that escapes and does not allow itself to be grasped, which may be those connected to the sense of death, or the effect of that navel through which the dream rests on the unknown. We are at the crossroads of several "dream factories", as René Kaës tells us, postulating a second navel in which "The dream feeds on the intersubjective mycelium and arises from the unconscious embedded in shared psychic space" (2002).

In search of new territories, we resort to myth, art, and fantasy which have the stuff that dreams and emotions are made of (Ginzburg, 2020). The amplification of the dream as a waking dream constitutes one of the pinnacles from which an in-depth examination of the use of dreams in clinical practice can begin.

I revisit my interrupted dream by changing language, using that of myth, like a journey into the underworld, the one narrated by Homer in the "Hymn to Demeter", the maternal goddess of the earth, of wheat, of seasons. Demeter's suffering over the abduction of her daughter Persephone by Hades is a cosmic sorrow. She abdicates her divine function and the earth becomes sterile; not even the gods of Olympus can oppose her, so Zeus intercedes and the god of the underworld must obey by letting Persephone return to earth, but not without first making her eat a pomegranate grain that will bind her forever to the underworld, where she will have to spend a third of the year, a period in which the earth will not produce fruit. Strong is the myth's reference to the nourishment of the bond of love and the famine due to its lack, which makes Demeter the most powerful of the Olympian gods. At the same time, drawing nourishment from the depths of the underworld creates an indissoluble bond, just as, through therapeutic processing, opening the doors of the unconscious leads to the discovery of new territories that will forever transform one's self-awareness.

By identifying the place of trauma with the underworld, reaching the patient in Hades means reaching the traumatic area ourselves and being able to experience it without being destroyed by it; an area belonging to the unrepressed unconscious, the deepest, archaic, which is intertwined and confused with the body itself.

To go where there is no formulation of experience, it is necessary to look for other languages of representation, through art, myth, dream. It is necessary, as Ferruta (2021) says, "to pave the way for other forms of unconscious communication between analyst and analysand", succeeding, through mythical and metaphorical narrative, to create internal resonances to give fullness to the elusive descriptions of unconscious dynamics.

Lastly, I would like to remind you, with one last dream I had the night after a first psychotherapy session, that descending into the unconscious underworld is not only terrifying but can also become creative and transformative.

Clinical example: A.

The young A.'s description of her life is more than a little evasive, her emotions do not find a natural way out, as when she says, slightly laughing, that she has kept some psychotropic drugs aside in order to be able, one day, to take them all at once; or even how she cannot express in any way her annoyance with her intrusive and controlling boss, showing, on the contrary, passiveness and acquiescence. A. was removed from her family, not by the social services, helpless spectators of a clogged bureaucracy, but by the intervention of a private association that she contacted. A. had two experiences of psychotherapy, but in one of these she was forced to listen to the therapist's accounts of her private life, to follow her precepts and suffer her criticism. Once again, she was alone.

When she leaves at the end of the session, she tells me "Thank you very much". Her gaze is firm, her voice is firm.

The same night I had this dream:

> A girl has stuck her head between the bars of a railing on a flight of steps, she cannot get out, in the attempt she injures herself, her body is heavy, she is in danger. I get closer, lift her up to support her body while helping her turn her head in the right direction. Finally, she manages to free herself and we hug each other.

On waking up, I immediately think of the dream and the patient. This time, an uninterrupted therapeutic function seems to have been possible, releasing a strong creative energy; one would have to reckon, in this case, not with the therapist's pain but with his narcissistic, omnipotent or manic aspects, perhaps even more difficult to observe. Pain and omnipotence, two polarities that live in the *dough* of the good bread on which the patient can, for a while, feed.

The therapist's body, the therapist's dreams, the amplification to other areas such as those of art, myths, literature, are new territories that in the therapeutic process the therapist makes available within himself and that the patient can explore by amplifying the possibility of self-understanding.

This requires a willingness on the part of the therapist to countertransference (Bollas, 1987), to his or her own continuous self-analysis, tolerating not knowing precisely what is being dealt with, until some hypothesis comes to the fore, and "Whoever would hasten to reproach me for this, please try to be more sincere than I am" (Freud, 1900–1901 [2001]). The aim is to be able to keep the patient, the images he or she arouses in us, and his or her contents inside for as long as is necessary for unconscious experiences in search of sharing to find the contact necessary for growth.

The therapist's dreams in supervision
Cristina Pratesi

An area of particular interest in the clinic and training of psychoanalytic psychotherapists concerns what can happen in supervision sessions. We know that in supervision in psychoanalytic psychotherapy, the supervisor's task is to stimulate the therapist to think, helping him not to conceive of his function as inspired by an obligation, but to value creativity, emotional closeness to patients, authenticity, spontaneity, reflection, intuition.

> The power of unconscious intuition that puts him in deep emotional contact with his patient ... tuning in, containing anxieties, creating an emotional field, maintaining sufficiently adequate tranquillity, using reverie ... giving time to emotions to manifest themselves, building a working alliance, creating trust, developing the observation of one's Ego, fortifying it by highlighting positive resources, represent the guidelines, the technique to be acquired and in essence the most appropriate ways to conduct ... a skilled supervision.
>
> (Romano Toscani, 2017)

It is therefore fundamental, as supervisors, not to pass judgement on what the therapist did or did not do or say in the session with the patient (which would undoubtedly only lead to mortification), not to transmit a rigid model, shaped by a superego, to conform to, but rather to help the trainee to realise his or her own, personal style, which represents the authentic essence of his or her being as a person.

The trainee must be helped to reflect on the conscious motivations that led him to carry out a certain type of intervention with the material brought in by the patient rather than another, so as to understand his own limitations, and also his own unconscious motivations, of which to become aware and on which to then work in his own personal analysis.

However, the fear that many trainee psychotherapists experience when starting a supervision is not always referred to, sometimes due to the trainee's image of the supervisor as a defender of dogma, committed to transmitting unchangeable theoretical and technical knowledge, fixed so, and ready to label everything that the trainee brings to him/her, exclusively as a reflection of the therapist's own difficulties that have not been sufficiently analysed, or as conflicts that he/she has not examined in the relationship with his/her patient.

Precisely the dream of a young therapist during his supervision can help us to illustrate and better understand how important, in psychoanalytic psychotherapy, the function of a supervisor is, who, makes it possible to experience, and thus learn, a flexible modality that encourages the trainee to maintain his own authenticity, so as to be able in turn to develop his patient's authenticity.

A student psychotherapist reports to his supervisor dreams he has had immediately after the supervision sessions, dreams which he rightly considers to be an integral part of his personal analysis, but also of his training. In one of these dreams, he is helping his mother-in-law with the household chores: he knows he has to be good, a good son-in-law who meets her expectations, but he feels he does it willingly.

He says that in the dream the house is cosy, warm, there is a calm, relaxed atmosphere. He comments that he knows he is very much in need of being welcomed, that he would not be able to talk, to tell the sessions to a supervisor he feels is rigid, judgemental, castrating. He is bothered by coercion, because he feels it is an obstacle to true understanding, both of the clinical material and of the nature of his therapeutic relationship with the patient.

The sense of fear, shame, sometimes even guilt on the part of young therapists often results in resistance, particularly with regard to countertransference dreams, which are rarely brought up in supervision, with the result that they are not discussed, understood and processed. But it is precisely the supervised work on these dreams – which are the product of the interaction of the patient's and the therapist's subjectivities – that makes the therapist aware of the patient's deeper, unconscious levels, of the indispensable symbolic elaboration of the projective identifications with which the patient communicates (Ogden, 1996).

It is in the interplay of cross-projections that there is also an experience that for a student therapist can be destabilising and therefore not communicable in supervision, for fear of having crossed a line, of having done something profoundly wrong, forbidden, and therefore of incurring reprobation, blame, criticism from the supervisor: I am referring to that particular situation that arises when the therapist dreams the same dream as the patient.[15]

The same young psychotherapist in training reports, in supervision, the dream of one of his patients, a beautiful girl in her thirties, describing her painful, unworked-through abandonment by her father when she was 6 years old. The girl dreams of joining him for the session: in the house where the patient is brought in, instead of in the office, there is a very informal and relaxed atmosphere, and the therapist tells her: "Now, instead of having the session, let's go for a walk!"

The night after this session with the patient, the therapist dreams that he is outside his analyst's office, waiting to go in for his own session. The analyst, however, tells him: "Let's not have a session, let's go for a walk!"

Beyond the aspects of exclusive relevance to the work in one's own personal analysis (and the young therapist's not so unconscious desire to know what his analyst would have done in his place in a similar situation), what is significant in this double dream, which also leads us to reflect on the concept of the "shared dream",[16] is the change of plan in the patient/psychotherapist relationship in the direction of greater intimacy, but also the request for authorisation to allow oneself greater freedom, as with a trip out of town. To be legitimised to allow oneself a pleasure, as well as having to be.

Through the countertransference dream, the therapist is then helped by the supervisor to better understand the need the patient expresses, to understand that he is impersonating unconscious parts of the patient that contact his receptive unconscious through projective identification, to recognise the point of interface, of interaction, where his psyche and that of the patient meet (Brown, 2004), to become aware "of sharing primitive mental passages, concrete, effective and meaningful as those experienced in dreams" (Bolognini, 2008). We know, in fact, that it is precisely when the patient's untransformed emotional experiences are too intense that the therapist's capacity for rêverie is "put in check" and the countertransference dream is produced (which in the relational perspective we prefer to call "the therapist's dream"). And it is exclusively through the work carried out by the therapist together with his or her supervisor that a rêverie is reactivated, like a four-handed sonata, an imaginative process as a couple, which allows the therapist to start using his or her unconscious again to "bring the patient into existence through dreams" (Ogden, 2016).

Also, in the situation presented, through the therapist's dream work, supervision allowed the young therapist-in-training to complete the way his mind is experiencing the patient, taking on the unacceptable parts of the patient herself and finding "symbols for what [she] cannot independently mentalise" (Brown, 2007).

Notes

1 I am referring to the different consideration of the mind-body relationship.
2 The psyche-soma is the sensory experience from which the mind takes shape:

> Given the necessary environmental conditions, the intellect is a specialised part of the general organisation of the integration of psyche and soma in the child. As such it does not exist separately but is the imaginative elaboration of somatic parts, feelings and functions, i.e. of physical life.
>
> (Winnicott, 1949)

3 Allan Schore (1994) believes that the personality and the individual, both in healthy and integrated development and in psychopathology, are formed precisely on the basis of those first neuro-psychobiological and affective connections between

caregiver and child, starting from the unconscious (i.e., not conscious) dictated by care and love, between the right hemisphere of one in connection with the right hemisphere of the other.

4 Freud, while appreciating their contents, opposed Rank's theorisations on birth trauma because they undermined the centrality of the Oedipus underlying development; but he is believed to have incorporated these findings into his later conceptualisation of anxiety.

5 Psychosomatic training course on the therapeutic relationship – Massimo Rosselli Psychosomatic Training Institute, Florence.

6 He states, "a primitive, pre-symbolic, sensory-dominant mode ... that generates the most basic forms of human experience" (Ogden, 1989).

7 The concepts of embodied self, embodied mind, embodiment, where different disciplines (phenomenology, neuroscience, psychoanalysis) seem to converge to really question, even in Western thought, the illusory separation of mind and body.

8 Film directed by James McTeigue (USA/Germany, 2005).

9 See Racker's (1968) notion of complementary countertransference.

10 Barale and Ferro state:

> [T]he hypothesis we propose is that 'countertransference dreams' perform a function of rearranging the analytic mental equipment and the fabric of relations between internal objects called into play in the dream work, of reconstituting spaces of accommodation and symbolisation, of reorganising the activity of the alpha function (we might say in Bionian terms). in conditions where these functions are particularly challenged. Fine-tuning and rearranging operations which do not only concern the relationship with that single patient who may appear in the dream, but often groups or tangles of patients or of aspects partly raised by the patients and partly coming from the analyst's endogenous origin; even complex tangles which the dream takes charge of rearticulating. Ultimately, reflection on these phenomena, precisely because of their particular evidence, may be of some use in attempting to describe certain general aspects of the analytic relationship that often remain 'in the background', in a dimension that functions, but which eludes thematisation: a dimension that concerns that general background of signification that is constituted by the work done by the dream thought.
>
> (1987)

11 "The analyst's unconscious contains the patient's unconscious" (Racker, 1968). In supervision, the supervisor contains therapist and patient.

12 The general definition of the concept of intersubjectivity in recent North American and European psychoanalytic dictionaries (IPA's *Inter-Regional Encyclopedic Dictionary of Psychoanalysis*, 2021) emphasises the reciprocal dynamic interaction between people, characterised by many facets and many levels, based on their subjective experiences (conscious, pre-conscious and/or unconscious) and a variety of mutually transformative interpenetration aspects in such encounters, both in the early stages of development and in psychoanalytic dialogue.

13 M. Little (1951) describes and valorises the communicative use of countertransference interpretations.

14 From a discussion with the members/psychotherapists of the ASPIG Association.

15 I sincerely thank Luca Ricci for allowing me to use his clinical material.

16 The function of rêverie that the psychotherapist performs with his patients, welcoming their dreams and dreaming himself, as Meltzer (1984) points out, also

seems to recall what Racamier expressed when he emphasised that "one never sleeps alone, but clutched to the body diffusely invested in the primitive mother" (1976). It is this maternal dimension of the primal dream-space that is the source of shared dreams. Pontalis (1986) also emphasises the experience of a common and shared intermediate area, a space of encounter and exchange, as reported by Kaës (2002).

References

Barale, F. and Ferro, A. (1987). Sofferenza mentale nell'analista e sogni di contro-transfert. *Rivista di Psicoanalisi*, 2: 219–233.

Bastianini, T., Ferruta, A. and Guerrini Degl'Innocenti, B. (2021). *Ascoltare con tutti i sensi. Estensioni del paradigma dell'ascolto psicoanalitico.* Rome: Giovanni Fioriti Editore.

Bollas, C. (1987). *The Shadow of the Object: Psychoanalysis of the Unthought Known.* London: Free Association Books.

Bolognini, S. (2002). *L'empatia psicoanalitica.* Turin: Bollati Boringhieri.

Bolognini, S. (2008). *Passaggi segreti. Teoria e tecnica della relazione interpsichica.* Turin: Bollati Boringhieri.

Bolognini, S. (2020). Riflessioni sulla pandemia. Available at: https://www.spiweb.it/wp content/uploads/2020/03/bolognini.pdf.

Bolognini, S. (2021). Paper presented at Congresso SPI, Inconscio, inconsci, 4–7 February 2021

Bonamimio, V. (2017). Clinical Winnicott: Traveling a Revolutionary Road. *The Psychoanalytical Quarterly*, 86(3): 609–626.

Borgogno, F., Luchetti, A., and Marino Coe, L. (2017). *Il pensiero psicoanalitico italiano. Maestri, idee e tendenze dagli anni '20 ad oggi.* Milan: FrancoAngeli.

Brown, L.J. (2004). The Point of Interaction, Mutuality, and an Aspect of the Analyst's Oedipus Conflict. *The Scandinavian Psychoanalytic Review*, 27: 34–42.

Ferenczi, S. (1958). *Journal clinique.* Paris: Payot.

Ferenczi, S. (1982). Confusion de langue entre les adultes et l'enfant. Le langage de la tendresse et de la passion. In S. Ferenczi, *Œuvres complètes*, vol. IV: *Psychanalyse: 1927–1933.* Paris: Payot.

Ferruta, A. (2011). "Wo Es war soll Ich werden" nel pensiero di Elvio Fachinelli. In N. Pirillo (ed.), *Elvio Fachinelli e la domanda della Sfinge. Tra psicoanalisi e pratiche filosofiche.* Naples: Liguori Editore.

Ferruta, A. (2020). Una riflessione sul pensiero di Fachinelli. *Psicoterapia Psicoanalitica*, 1: 109–118.

Ferruta, A. (2021). Ermes. Comunicare con le dimensioni inconsce della psiche. *Rivista di Psicoanalisi*, LXVII(2): 347–362.

Freud, S. (1900–1901 [2001]). The Interpretation of Dreams (I). The Interpretation of Dreams (II) and On Dreams. In J. Strachey (ed.), *The Standard Edition of the Complete Psychological Works of Sigmund Freud*, vol. IV (*1900*) and vol .V (*1900–1901*). London: Hogarth Press.

Freud, S. (1915–1917 [2002]). Introduction to Psychoanalysis. In J. Strachey (ed.), *The Standard Edition of the Complete Psychological Works of Sigmund Freud*, vol. XV. London: Hogarth Press.

Freud, S. (1938 [2001]). Splitting of the Ego in the Process of Defence. In J. Strachey (ed.), *The Standard Edition of the Complete Psychological Works of Sigmund Freud*, vol. XXIII *(1937–1939)*. London: Hogarth Press.

Ginzburg, A. (2020). *La stoffa di cui sono fatti i sogni e le emozioni*. Rome: Alpes Italia.

Hautmann, G. (1965). Un esempio di controidentificazione proiettiva. In G. Hautmann, *Funzione analitica e mente primitiva*. Pisa: Edizioni ETS.

IPA (2021). *Inter-Regional Encyclopedic Dictionary of Psychoanalysis*. Available at: www.ipa.world (accessed 3 May 2021).

Kaës, R. (2002). *La polyphonie du rêve. L'expérience onirique commune et portage*. Paris: Dunod.

Little, M. (1951). Counter-Transference and the Patient's Response to It. *The International Journal of Psychoanalysis*, 32: 32–40.

Meltzer, D. (1984). *Dream-Life: A Re-Examination of the Psycho-Analytical Theory and Technique*. Glen Lyon, Perthshire: Clunie Press.

Meltzer, D. (1992). *The Claustrum: An Investigation of Claustrophobic Phenomena*. Glen Lyon, Perthshire: Clunie Press.

Mucci, C. (2020). *Corpi borderline. Regolazione affettiva e clinica dei disturbi di personalità*. Milan: Raffaello Cortina.

Nissim Momigliano, L. (1983). Analista e paziente al lavoro: una sonata a quattro mani. In L. Nissim Momigliano, *L'ascolto rispettoso. Scritti psicoanalitici*. Milan: Raffaello Cortina.

Nissim Momigliano, L. (1984). Due persone che parlano in una stanza. Una ricerca sul dialogo analitico. *Rivista di Psicoanalisi*, 30: 1–17.

Ogden, T.H. (1989). *The Primitive Edge of Experience*. London: Routledge.

Ogden, T.H. (1996). Reconsidering Three Aspects of Psychoanalytic Technique. *International Journal of Psychoanalysis*, 77: 883–899.

Ogden, T.H. (2005). This Art of Psychoanalysis: Dreaming Undreamt Dreams and Interrupted Cries. *International Journal of Psychoanalysis*, 85: 857–877.

Ogden, T.H. (2016). *Reclaiming Unlived Life: Experiences in Psychoanalysis*. New York: Routledge.

Pontalis, J.B. (1986). *L'Amour des commencements*. Paris: Gallimard.

Racamier, P.C. (1976). Rêve et psychose: rêve ou psychose? *Revue Française de Psychoanalyse*, XL.

Racker, H. (1968). *Transference and Countertransference*. New York: International Universities Press.

Romano Toscani, R. (2017). *Conversazione a due voci. Note sulla supervisione*. Milan: FrancoAngeli.

Schore, A.N. (1994). *Affect Regulation and the Origin of the Self: The Neurobiology of Emotional Development*. Hillsdale, NJ: Lawrence Erlbaum Associates.

Semi, A. (2017). Il transfert e le comunicazioni inconsce: controtransfert, teorie e narcisismo dell'analista. In F. Borgogno, A. Luchetti and L. Marino Coe (eds), *Il pensiero psicoanalitico italiano. Maestri, idee e tendenze dagli anni '20 ad oggi*. Milan: FrancoAngeli.

Winnicott, D.W. (1949). Mind and its Relation to the Psyche-Soma. In D.W. Winnicott, *Collected Papers: Through Paediatrics to Psycho-Analysis*. London: Hogarth Press.

Chapter 6

Patients unable to dream

Alfredina Fiori and Cristina Pratesi

In our practices we increasingly welcome patients whose requests lead us to take note of a marked change in pathology. Narcissistic type organisations appear today to be transversal to many pathologies and personality structures.

Some patients present states of suffering that manifest themselves with great frequency and in a repetitive manner through somatisations or in any case with an attention directed almost exclusively at daily life, where the body and physical pain often appear to be the only indicators of the emotional content and psychic suffering, wordless interlocutors that do not allow the patient to make sense of what is happening to him. It therefore becomes necessary for the therapist to work tirelessly to construct a shared language and code of reading, helping the patient to transform suffering into a narrative: just as the pathology of patients is changing, it is therefore just as indispensable to diversify the modes of reception and therapeutic work.

In psychoanalytic psychotherapy, more than anywhere else, it is in fact evident how the fundamental transformative factor consists in the quality of the therapist's mental functioning, in the relational instant of the session, thanks to that process that W. Bion called "waking dream thinking" (1962). which evokes in the therapist's mind "the patient's internal states (and his own) in the form of vivid and precise visual images" (Ferro, 2008).

The therapist brings to the encounter his capacity for waking dream thoughts, which he transmits to the patient from time to time, not necessarily through interpretations, but rather through his own gifts of empathy, containment, tolerance and expectation so that he can refine over time his own capacity to access the dream dimension.[1] In the therapeutic relationship, one thus builds the possibility of being in the mind of the Other and grasping, in a mutual dialogue, the representation of oneself in the Other.

We know that the Ego of the narcissistic type cannot always tolerate intrusion into its own secret history; it does not accept being the object of exploration but only the subject, and therefore the exploration and sharing of the symbolic dimension can be experienced as a violation of the frontiers of its own life space. Not everything can be said directly and the therapist must respect distances and use the necessary mediations to protect the patient-

DOI: 10.4324/9781032673721-7

therapist relationship, leaving a possible interpretation in silence and suspension. This would in fact assume the dimension of aggressive intrusion, insisting on a dogmatic exploration that does not tolerate doubt.

Discovering the presence of an internal and unknown world, discovering spaces and images capable of profoundly affecting, discovering contents and emotions that can overturn and profoundly change the usual world, awakens and sets in motion an anxiety that cannot be tolerated.

The reflection we would like to share here is how many patients can lead the therapist to fear that they are unable to escape from a vicious circle, from a pathology that does not allow them to build a psychic space. Bion would say that these patients are not able to dream.

Psychotherapy thus becomes the tool that helps the patient build the capacity to dream. The therapist's task is carried out in a similar way to that of a parent or caregiver who helps to activate an imaginative function that is essential for a child's psychic health. The absence or blockage of this function causes existential impasses and claustrophobic pain, which underlie many psychic disorders. The recovery of imaginative freedom and meaning is a foundational experience that is closely tied to the state of health (Cresti and Suman, 2014).

Bion tells us that the patient who is unable to transform his emotional experiences into alpha elements, cannot even dream, whereas the ability to dream seems to preserve the personality from a virtually psychotic state (Bion, 1962). In this perspective, the capacity to dream, then, stands as a "watershed" between a psychic functioning oriented towards symbolisation (the neurotic part of the personality) and a psychic functioning oriented towards the evacuation of tensions and therefore incapable of constructing representations and producing dream thoughts (the psychotic part) (Guarnieri, 2003).

Telling a dream is a way of discovering oneself, of opening up to the other and establishing contact and exchange with the world. This can be felt as threatening, if not as impossible, in order not to break the protective autistic shell of a psyche with a narcissistic structure, which can only accept its own image and cancel everything that is other than itself (Kohut, 1971). Dreaming is a way of expressing oneself and communicating with oneself and with the other, but to truly be with the other, one must first be with oneself. Also according to Masud Khan (1972). who reprises the Freudian concept of dreamwork, dreaming is an activity closely linked to the ego's ability to use symbolisation, through which the processing of unconscious contents in the dream is realised.

And, therefore, what to do when a patient does not bring dream material and does not make accessible, as T. Ogden (2003; 2009) says, the "lived experiences" to the unconscious thought processes, transforming thought into emotional experience (from the conscious to the unconscious)? It is necessary to help the patient to dream up a previously undreamable experience, in other words, to give a symbolic personal meaning to the lived experience. To lead the patient to reflect on the relationship and his life, to understand its emotional meaning by recovering those split-off aspects that cannot be dreamt but only relived and processed through the therapist's "talking" that becomes thought and mind that contain it.

Cases

A borderline patient

An example of this is a case recounted by S. Fano Cassese (2010). This is the case of a woman who had suffered various abandonments and separations in childhood and had built up a defensive shell based on her social position, which she had managed to conquer through hard sacrifice. Although the patient immediately gave me the impression that she wanted to manage the therapy and control me, I underestimated the extent of this attitude, as I later realised in the transference relationship, which oscillated between idealisation and aggressive attacks, continuous agitation, intrusive behaviour and sometimes paranoid experiences, with a tendency to role reversal. From the beginning of therapy, I felt fascinated by this person, beautiful and intelligent, who challenged me and with whom I felt affinities, linked to some of my personal aspects. Initially, my tendency to identify with her perhaps led me to steer my interpretations in a certain direction. In fact, I felt she was very fragile and defenceless, under her – sometimes arrogant – veneer, but she refused all my attempts to get in touch with this childish "orphan" part of her, accusing me of not having understood anything about her, that she was a successful woman, who held a prestigious position. I feared that breaking through her split-off part could be dangerous, with the risk of a psychotic break-down. To overcome the impasse I was in, I decided to avoid any interpretation and to work differently. I thought that I had to be a point of reference for her, to help her find a more authentic sense of Self and that to do this I had to use my own points of reference, even accepting a more "equal" or "symmetrical" relationship. A more fruitful period of work began in which I felt more relaxed, I could then discuss literature, art, etc. with her, but also her relational life, and then her childhood memories and first dreams, which she brought to the session after several months. I had the impression that these "conversations" had opened up a glimmer of certain experiences from her past that had hitherto been unthinkable, and that a process of transforming the experiences into "daydreams" in the Bionian sense, i.e., into something emotional and symbolisable which can be thought (Bion, 1962).

To illustrate her technique, Fano Cassese refers to what D. Meltzer (1973) called "inspired interpretations" in which, within an equal relationship with the patient, there is a personal involvement of the analyst. Meltzer thought they should be given at the end of the analysis when the analyst is preparing to increasingly become the patient's real object. Fano Cassese, on the other hand, finds them useful in all those cases and in all those moments of the therapy when the therapist has to help the patient dream: "Talking as dreaming" is, states Ogden (2009). a form of improvisation, a conversation, which can range over any subject, in which the analyst participates in the patient's "undreamed dreams" with his own free associations and self-reflections, thus helping him to "dream himself into existence".

Adriana[2]

So, what about Adriana who started psychotherapy at the age of 50 and does not dream? The feeling of estrangement that has accompanied her from pre-adolescence onwards, like a sense of non-existence, of emotional detachment and estrangement from what is happening to her and in her world, is the reason that led her to begin a therapeutic journey that will be long and very tiring.

The second child of a very poor, an affective violent and totally uneducated family, which sent her to work at the age of 11 as an apprentice and then as a factory worker, Adriana spent her life conforming to models that she felt were imposed on her: she married, had children, took care of the house, while working in the factory with gruelling shifts.

Dreams never appear in the session; Adriana says to the therapist: "I never dream. You say that everyone dreams, but I really don't know if I can't dream or if I don't remember. In my opinion, I don't dream." The concrete account of the events of the week fills her sessions, which for years run flat, without ever a single cry: only, sometimes, nervous giggles, very irritating for the therapist, who perceives them as so out of place that she wonders whether the patient has a cognitive deficit. There is no possibility of access to symbolisation: her world and her very existence can only be concrete, extremely simple, at the limits of norm/insufficiency.

The patient started to write a diary in the third year of therapy which led to a decisive change. Initially, she reported on the course of therapy through the account of her feelings for her therapist, which she sent to the National Diary Archive in Pieve Santo Stefano, with a request for anonymity. The diary did not win the prize, but it received a special mention, which prompted her to continue writing and participating in literary competitions at a regional level, in which she often came first.

She brings her short stories to the therapist; they are very short and written in a simple but lucid and passionate style, which become the material of the sessions, because it is only through the stories, always and only set in her childhood years, that Adriana can give voice to her emotions, to her feelings, otherwise "frozen" within her, impossible to reach, of which she is still ashamed to speak in the first person. Through the analysis of the stories, as if they were the equivalent of dreams, her anger, her envy, her feared – but never acted upon – homosexuality can find "shelter" at last.

It was not until the end of the sixth year of therapy that her first dream appeared:

> I was in a house that I knew was mine. Suddenly the door swung open violently and a gigantic man entered, black-skinned, dirty and with tattered clothes, who wordlessly, with an overbearing and arrogant manner, threw himself on my bed. I complain to the woman who was behind him, scolding her for not stopping him from entering and behaving like a master.

Through various passages, she is able to associate the dream with the moment of her father's return from prison, the father whom she had never met, and who had destroyed, with his intrusive presence, "the all-female paradise" in which she had been born and lived until the age of 3, cared for and pampered by her maternal grandmother and her father's aunts, very old and spinsterish, who all lived nearby, while her mother, rigid and with a frozen femininity, not at all affectionate, worked. From that moment on, everything had changed forever. At the end of the session, Adriana told me: "I have lost a lot by not dreaming: it is so satisfying to know what is hidden in a dream that seems so bizarre … I am always in time to make amends."

Marzia[3]

In another patient, Marzia, the effort to dominate anger leads her to narcissistic actions and behaviour and to systematically develop somatic symptoms, some of them quite disabling, though fortunately in a transitory way. Accepting her depressive dimension will allow her, after many years of psychotherapy, to create – through long-silenced dream production – the possibility of listening to her emotional space and to control her aggressiveness and destructive anxiety, building a bridge between body and mind.

Marzia, whose mother had suffered from severe depression, had started a previous psychotherapy to treat the panic attacks she was subjected to, but interrupted it with a violent verbal clash; she recounts that she felt "kicked out" by the therapist who accused her of activating anger. She now asks for support because she feels unable to be a mother; she says she never knows what rules and boundaries to keep with her children. She then speaks of the horror vacui that forces her to always take care of something, to fill herself with commitments so as not to feel her inner emptiness. She states that she has a recurring dream that has accompanied her for some time: the house, that is, having to fix, clear, arrange houses. For a long time, however, she has been unable to dream, and throughout the first three years of therapy she continues to have no dreams at all, while copious somatic symptoms flourish, ranging from the appearance of widespread and intensive tics to admissions to the emergency ward for illnesses that appear suddenly and violently, but fortunately with an ultimately mild outcome. However, she cannot accept the idea that this physical malaise is connected to an emotional criticality.

Together we observe that the somatic symptoms serve to calm her down without feeling guilty, allowing her to explore the emotional dimension and give substance to her creativity. Encouraged by a friend, she resumed her artistic activity to the point of staging a personal exhibition which proved to be successful. After three years of psychotherapy and a week before the exhibition, she brings her first dream "the usually dark and cluttered house now has a window and can be put in order". She then opens the "dream notebook" and, at least once a month, brings a dream. The dreams alternate with a production of somatic symptoms, progressively less violent, and an unstoppable artistic production that makes her fill furniture, drawers and every space in the house with her creations. After many more years of meeting and working together, Marzia recently brought a dream, once again of a house:

> In the kitchen, I open a wall unit and discover a large empty space. Elated by the discovery, I regret not having discovered it sooner. At the end of this space, a small shelf with stacked reams of paper on it, in order. I think I will be able to put all my works here, perhaps there might even be enough space for a piece of furniture to share with my brother.

Artistic creation, as an expression of the unspeakable, of thoughts that cannot be expressed in words, enables Marzia to accept her depressive position and to control her aggression, or rather to be able to tolerate it without necessarily acting it out towards herself or others. It allows her to be able to think that she is not necessarily guilty of the sufferings of the people she asks for help from (her depressed mother, the therapist she angered and harmed, etc.). Her way of communicating is conveyed through the physicality of her emotional experience: her emotions become visible and embodied in an artistic work that performs a function of containment, and at the same time, makes it possible for her to get in touch with her narcissistic and depressive aspects. Through her "works", the patient reaches the symbolic dimension that creates a bridge between body and mind, which she still needs to cross in both directions.

Conclusion

In conclusion, we observe how, in the clinical cases narrated, the world of creativity becomes a mediation between dreaming and waking in a blurred space and time that allows one to simultaneously think and create in different dimensions. The creative act is a way of memory surfacing recreating a new image of the world, and the dream is the gateway that separates from an invisible world. Narcissistic forces are directed, through creative work, towards a new, higher "self-object" (Kohut, 1971). thanks to the liberation of creative capacities and the release of narcissistic tensions which had previously been a serious threat to affective and physical health.

The dream is, therefore, a project, an itinerary, a movement towards a possible stage of a journey, and the therapist is the bridge that allows the passage between bodily reality and psyche, between sleep and wakefulness: it is the audience that witnesses and gives meaning to the dream scene and its representation (Resnik, 1987).

Notes

1 As Ferro reminds us, "the need to construct a place for thinking thoughts, before the contents can be fully given, also applies to dreaming" (1999).
2 The case was treated by C. Pratesi.
3 The case was treated by A. Fiori.

References

Bion, W.R. (1962). *Learning from Experience*. London: Karnac Books.
Cresti, L. and Suman, A. (2014). *La psicoterapia psicoanalitica attuale: fattori terapeutici non-interpretativi*. Paper presented at the National Scientific Day, SIEFPP, Rome (unpublished text).
Fano Cassese, S. (2010). L'interpretazione ispirata e parlare come sognare. Available at: www.spi.firenze.it/l-interpretazione-ispirata-e-parlare-come-sognare-silvia-fano-cassese/ (accessed 8 November 2020.).
Ferro, A. (1999). *La Psicoanalisi come letteratura e terapia*. Milan: Raffaello Cortina.
Ferro, A. (2008). *Rêveries*. Turin: Antigone.
Guarnieri, M. (2003). Vedere, pensare, sognare. In F. Riolo (ed.), *L'analisi dei sogni. Gli scritti del 6° Colloquio di Palermo*. Milan: FrancoAngeli.
Kahn, M. (1972). Use and Abuse of Dreams in Psychic Experience. In M. Kahn, *The Privacy of the Self*. London: Hogarth Press.
Kohut, H. (1971). *The Analysis of the Self*. London: Hogarth Press.
Meltzer, D. (1973). L'interpretazione di routine e l'interpretazione ispirata. In D. Meltzer, *La comprensione della bellezza*. Turin: Loescher.
Ogden, T.H. (2003) On Not Being Able to Dream. *International Journal of Psychoanalysis*, 84: 17–30.
Ogden, T.H. (2009). *Rediscovering Psychoanalysis: Thinking and Dreaming, Learning and Forgetting*. London: Routledge.
Resnik, S. (1987). *The Theatre of the Dream*. London: Routledge.

Chapter 7

Adaptations of technique in the psychotherapy of borderline patients

Corrado D'Agostini

The new organisation of psychopathology described in the *Psychodynamic Diagnostic Manual* (PDM), by shifting the focus from the symptom to the person's mental functioning, made it possible to observe personality disorders from a different perspective that inevitably ended up being affected in psychotherapeutic work by the *Diagnostic and Statistical Manual of Mental Disorders'* (DSM) proposed framework. In particular, the borderline problematic broke away from the simplified definition useful for the most striking symptomatologic conditions, and instead became part of the broader panorama of problems relating to the construction and functioning of identity. Patients with a non-integrated sense of identity currently account for a significant proportion of those who come to clinical observation while, at the same time, deficiencies in the sense of identity constitute the typical feature of much of the psychological problematic that the PDM defines as borderline personality organisation. Their treatment requires a psychotherapeutic technique that is significantly different from the traditional one that, in the psychodynamic perspective, finds a central element in interpretation.

Usually the term borderline is attributed to turbulent patients who are frequently admitted to psychiatric emergency rooms due to their emotional and behavioural intemperance, whereas in PDM-2 borderline organisation is not referred to as a nosological class in its own right but refers to patients who present deficiencies in the construction and functioning of a stable identity. Psychotic, borderline, neurotic and normal organisation thus do not constitute coherent evolutionary personality classes with clear-cut boundaries, but dynamic areas of mental functioning at different evolutionary levels, with partially open boundaries and modes of thinking related to the person's condition in the here and now.

The term borderline that dated back to the studies of Adolph Stern (1938) and Robert Knight (1953; 1954) was later taken up by Otto Kernberg (1967; 1975) who proposed the concept of Borderline Personality Organisation.[1] Kernberg's idea appeared when it was presented as too general and was further defined by Roy Grinker (1968) who identified its four typical aspects.[2]

DOI: 10.4324/9781032673721-8

The concept of borderline went from being an *organisation*, to being seen as a *syndrome* (Grinker, 1968). and then with the work of Spitzer and Endicott (1979) became a *personality disorder* in the DSM III of 1980. The focus on the disorder was not theoretical but was motivated by the fact that what in previous decades had been a very rare picture, in the USA at the end of the last century, had turned out to be extremely frequent with a prevalence of 2–3% of the general population and 25% of the total among hospitalised patients (Gunderson and Ridolfi, 2001). Grinker (1968) hypothesised that borderline psychopathology could be the result of the social and economic changes that occurred during the twentieth century, where previously the burden of manual labour and less leisure time, the demands of survival in a context of lesser well-being, had functioned as structuring elements to prevent or contain these psychopathological aspects.

After DSM III, subsequent editions confirmed the symptomatologic characteristics of borderline disorder as a personality disorder, while the aim of linking the disorder to its biological components did not come to fruition.

In 2006, the PDM was published, whose ideological proposal was *to actually observe psychic phenomena and adapt the psychodynamic method to the phenomena, rather than the other way around.* The PDM took from Kernberg the notion of Personality Organisation (P-axis) consisting of four components consisting of: (1) the sense of Identity, i.e., the ability to see oneself in a complex, stable and accurate manner; (2) the quality of object relations; (3) the level of defences; and (4) the reality examination. Attention was diverted from the symptom to focus on the function of the internal components of thought and the ability to exercise them. It is this functioning-based approach that gives the PDM greater heuristic value. Mention was made of the function of the structuring elements whose deficiency characterises borderline organisation. To be exercised, this function requires the capacity and integration of various brain structures.

In the mature personality, the ability to see oneself in a complex, stable and accurate manner with intimate, continuous and fulfilling object relationships characterises the sense of identity. The ability to integrate one's own identity, the ability to regulate internal experience, and self-observation skills characterise post-adolescent mental functioning.

In this regard, Gabbard, following the psychoanalytic tradition, spoke of splitting in observing the inability of borderlines to integrate positive and negative capacities in themselves and others, and observes that these people, due to splitting, are unable to integrate libidinal and aggressive aspects in their view of others and themselves, and thus suffer from mentalisation difficulties.

We can ask ourselves, in the light of the data that has emerged in recent years, whether these deficits can be attributed to a defence mechanism such as splitting or to a lack of integration capacity. These patients do not have a continuous tone vision of the sense of self fragmented by splits but seem to have a sense of identity formed by many islands of the self, separated as an archipelago, where areas and modes of thought have remained distant from the others, without a basic unifying structure.

If we consider the way these people speak, they are often unable to structure a discourse in a continuous manner, starting with the subject and then proceeding to the endpoint. They also show a certain difficulty in accessing the symbol, where the very etymology of the word indicates the ability to put together elements placed on different conceptual planes.

Far from being theoretical, the question of an insular view points towards different therapeutic strategies, in which this unrealised unifying condition ideally stands as the focus of therapeutic work.

G. Adler (1985) emphasised the inability of the borderline to make contact with a stable and comforting internal object due to an inconsistent or insufficient maternal function. In this view, the borderline patient, in his inability to exercise an evocative object memory, would be in search of object-self functions exercised by external figures.

Over the last few decades, the contributions of research using functional magnetic resonance imaging have confirmed that traumatic conditions, neglect and overall lack of synchronisation with the care figure are likely to generate physiological and anatomical changes in the child's brain. However, the link between these and the loss of the ability to regulate affect is now widely established (Shore, 2003), and how the disorganised-disoriented insecure attachment style, which is observed in abused and neglected children, anticipates later problems with affective regulation and the ability to cope with stress (Battle et al., 2004).

Beebe, Lachmann, and Jaffe (1997) examined patterns of mother-child interaction and their relevance to the pre-symbolic origins of self and object representations. Focusing on self and object representation, they highlighted how characteristic patterns of self and interaction regulation are formed on early interaction structures; it is these that provide an important basis for emergent self and object representations.

In children who have had deficient or disturbed interactions with the caregiver figure, the emotions will suffer and will not be integrated into consciousness, being constructively placed in the context of identity; they will be unmanageable and may give rise to impulsive or expulsive distress behaviour.

In the right hemisphere, experiences of neglect, abuse or stress, suffered emotionally, cannot be cognitively reorganised by the left hemisphere in order to be remembered. The left hemisphere only completes its primitive organisation around the age of 3, and traumatic experiences remain embedded in non-cognitive content that can only be expressed at the level of visceral experiences or unthought-actions. They are therefore destined to be part of the a-temporal, pre-symbolic and pre-verbal implicit memory. That memory constitutes what Mancia (1994; 2003) has defined as the unrepressed unconscious.[3]

These are the mental conditions that, whether or not combined with other genetic and environmental factors, are likely to constitute, in adolescence, pictures that can be traced in their clinical expression to personality disorders and specifically to a borderline personality organisation.

Experiences of abandonment or those that emotionally exceed the child's capacity for absorption, not finding symbolic and metaphorical expression, cannot be historicised and thus generate an absence of identity. It is to be assumed that this state of mind is close to what adult patients will later refer to as a sense of emptiness, derealisation and depersonalisation. The emotional overload that is not adequately metabolised and externalised through the historicizing functions of narration and representation, remains a prisoner of the unrepressed unconscious memory of the right orbitofrontal cortex that shows its deficit with an altered control of aggressive, impulsive, affective expression, sexual, eating and substance-taking behaviour.

This does not directly interfere with the person's intellectual level, but it certainly alters the possibilities of effective interaction in the social context. Affective dysregulation limits the possibility of resonance and integration with the emotional and operational context of the environment in which the subject is found. A mentalisation deficit appears. It is not appropriate to dwell on the techniques of mentalisation here today, but since borderline functioning can be characterised by conditions ranging from a slight momentary deficit in the capacity for integration to severe and constant destructuring, the intervention must be modulated accordingly. According to Bateman, Fonagy and Allen (2009), in situations of high emotional intensity of the patient, with a low level of mentalisation, interventions based on support and empathy are appropriate, to then move over time, when the level is characterised by reduced emotionality, progressively towards basic mentalisation with interventions involving the transference relationship. Franco De Masi (2013) in a report entitled "Borderline: a patient without an unconscious?" observed:

> If in these patients the function of the dynamic unconscious is deficient, it is not possible to give them interpretations of a symbolic type that presuppose a correspondence between manifest and repressed content, between conscious and unconscious ... While transference interpretation is for a long time impractical, it is instead much more useful to use descriptive intrapsychic interpretations of psychic functioning to help the patient develop those intuitive functions that he lacks.

Many authors (Gunderson, Links, Gabbard) insist that borderline patients require more structuring of therapy than other types of patients and recommend paying close attention to roles, goals, boundaries and concrete aspects of the setting. If this is not done, dynamic therapies may, in spite of themselves, increase the patient's anxiety levels. This is a risk not taken by cognitive-behavioural therapies, which are, by their nature, considerably structured.

Thus, the central element of therapy with patients who have an integration defect is containment and setting, but what setting? Bolognini (2008), regarding the setting, describes its *primary function as an agent of self-cohesion* identifying it "as an original restraining and regulative element … a structuring therapeutic factor capable of inducing long-term structural transformations, especially in patients who have not had a primary regulative experience".

The setting contains within itself a composite set of therapeutic elements, with its normative device intrinsically structured according to the paternal code, but also with its implicitly maternal nature. But which father and which mother? Not a standard codification suitable for all, but an element of recognition and growth that modulates, adapts flexibly to the process of emotional and cognitive growth and structuring.

Bolognini alludes to this again in *Secret Passages*, referring to the subtle emotional ties of the couple, in which an intrinsic reciprocal recognition between therapist and patient is therefore required, a reciprocal capacity for attraction, with the therapist's willingness to modulate certain elements of the relationship in the light of an *instinctuality* that, far from being wild, secure in a long discipline, now is absorbed to the point of being part of the very structure of the mind, and can be forgotten in order to be substantially reconstructed afterwards, similar to itself, but not necessarily identical. A silent container in which reciprocal proxemics, movements, mimicry, sounds, then voices, then the articulation of discourse, find space to be heard and reorganised in a musical sequence that tends towards the construction of a two-voice composition. In the construction of this score, the formulation of the contract, the structuring of the setting and the modalities of interaction may therefore require variable times and modes.

The arrangement implicitly contains a series of communications that do not only come through the therapist's awareness or the patient's feelings, but also through implicit contents of the two members of the couple. An arrangement, therefore, that, again, can only partly rely on the indications of the structured technique.

This is reminiscent of Beebe and Lachmann (2002; 2003), within the relational perspective, who argue that if the implicit and gestural modes of communication in psychotherapy are not taken into account, only half of what happens in the therapeutic encounter can be addressed.

The natural tendency to apply the reciprocal use of metaphor or the expression of certain concepts through mental images are some of the elements that can favour the construction of an imaginative language proper to the therapeutic couple. For example, during a session with a patient who was having difficulties in achieving a better definition of her own identity, it happened that both the patient and I lingered in an unusually long silence. For no apparent reason my gaze had lingered for a few minutes on the green pullover worn by the patient, who later informed me that she had silently thought of a yellow jacket of hers. Perhaps that mutual dwelling on the colour of a garment alluded to the search in our minds for a primitive mode of identity, perceived with a common sensory modality.

One may wonder whether the implicit contents in the couple's mind, and even more so those in the therapist's mind, are not a discriminating element for the success of this type of psychotherapy and whether these contents of the unconscious also determine the enactment in the session and in the course of therapy. We understand here in the term enactment what the work by Maria Ponsi (2012a) differentiated from acting-out, to bring it to the meaning of unconscious enactment of implicit contents of the couple's mind. For Ponsi (2012b). enactments, i.e., the continuous flow of micro-actions that accompany the verbal exchange between patient and therapist, are:

> ordinary occurrences that continually run through the patient-analyst relationship – occurrences that are not only inevitable, but also ubiquitous, since the dimension of action, or inter-action, is an intrinsic part of the analytic process. In this perspective, enactments would be like the tip of the iceberg, the most evident one, of this continuous interactive flow.

According to Shore (2012):

> Enactments are the expression of a dysregulation and re-actualisation of a traumatic experience through an implicit, right-brain-to-right-brain communication in which the patient's vulnerability interacts with the analyst's emotional availability ... The therapy no longer aims, as in classical psychoanalysis, at the conquest of the unconscious by the consciousness; the goal is rather the transformation and integration into the self of dissociated mental-cerebral areas through the regulation of affect ... In this perspective, enactment is the spearhead of a therapeutic action that brings to the fore what was previously in the background: the relationship.

But then, it seems to be clear that, with these patients, the characteristics and tools of the therapist's mind cannot be present in everyone equally and determine the success or failure of the therapeutic work.

Thus, personality characteristics take on a prominent role, since only when the relationship is expressed in a context of stable understanding, and a sufficient level of idealisation on the part of the patient has been achieved, do feelings of emptiness begin to become less dismaying, while the therapist helps in the construction of an internal framework of thought, in which the patient recognises himself and can place the fabric of his own rational acquisitions and a better relationship with his emotions.

This attunement is necessary because it is not enough for the patient to learn to relate better to internal and external objects, but also because he must be able to make sense of what he does. It is precisely this absence of meaning that causes the sense of emptiness.

Only after a certain amount of sense and directionality has been acquired, and a habit of collaboration and an expressive and engaging state of mind have stabilised, can the therapist even cautiously begin to offer some interpretation. Without these conditions, on the other hand, the use of interpretation is not appropriate and the therapist must use other therapeutic tools, such as, as we have shown, containment of the setting, gestural communication, including one's own personality. This is also why, in some respects, the therapist is well advised to offer partial identifications to which the patient can initially conform.

In this regard, we conclude with an enlightening reflection by Gunderson and Ridolfi (2001):

> Many therapists are not suitable for borderline patients. Thus it may be that Kernberg's or Linehan's success in cognitive-behavioural therapy with these patients can be attributed neither to their theories nor to their training. Perhaps the secret lies in what has been disparagingly referred to as the non-specific components of their offerings. Both Kernberg and Linehan are charismatic people. They are authoritative: they express confidence, lucidity, decisiveness and certainty ... both of them welcome the patient's emotional intensity or lability in a direct way, with a firm emotional intensity that is absolutely peculiar. Both convey to the patient the emotional perception that they are present, involved and unbreakable ... Kernberg's or Linehan's patients, I believe, are confident that their opinions, judgements or decisions will be heard and answered. What Swenson (1989) succinctly rendered as the feeling of being "emotionally contained." Attentive, provocative and sensitive: it is my opinion that these same qualities distinguish those who are excellent therapists for borderline patients.

A therapeutic experience in a borderline case

F.R., 32 years old, had struck me from the very first meeting because, instead of telling me why he had asked to see me, he had started insistently observing his surroundings, asking in detail what my professional qualifications were. To my invitation to talk about what had led him to me, he had responded by lamenting the fact that for the past ten years or so his life had been chronically dragging on between the fear of going mad with fears and fantasies of suicide, feelings of boredom and insignificance, and the desire and fear of leaving his partner whom he could not say whether he loved or not. He was frightened, however, by the possibility that she might leave him. He was also tormented by a series of "feelings and moods" that he could not describe while at the same time fearing to do so, because – he said – they might become more real. Constantly restless, mentally and physically, as I watched him, he could not sit still in the small chair in front of me. It was natural for him to try to peer into my identity, while I did not have to go into the depths of his emotions. Other previous therapists had tried to do this before he abandoned them. The tormenting times of his early adolescence, shattered by his father's severe financial hardship, represented a spectre that he feared might manifest itself again. Each sentence never managed to conclude its expressive cycle, because the discourse derailed, impulsively driven by new emotional emergencies, which in turn ended before they had been sufficiently recognised and described.

The initial interviews led to the identification of a borderline personality organisation in which the various aspects of identity, disrupted by unmanageable and indigestible emotional events, had not found adequate integration. F.R. asked me to immediately accept, understand and dissolve his fears without elaborating on them. The concepts of association and construction were unknown to him and he rejected any hypothesis with annoyance.

For my part, I thought it was my job to help him build bridges and lines of communication, so that the islands that made up the lagoon of his way of thinking were integrated with each other and acquired a sense of continuity, while he was uniquely absorbed in dealing with the emotion or sensation he was feeling at the time. He was immersed in the feeling of continuous suffering; a stable general condition of anxiety. The primitive feeling of care and trust was unknown to him; also music, the sound of which would have been suitable to comfort possible traumatic events such as those that occurred to the patient in his father's affairs. F.R.'s taunts and wails suggested to me a cry that demanded attention to him. It was appropriate to listen and remain silent, waiting for time to evoke the right emotions.

As with anorexic girls, in borderline organisations and in cases where there is a defect of individuation, it is not the interpretations that change the picture and favour the growth of the self, but the establishment of a deep feeling of primitive, instinctive acceptance. Something that derives above all from the implicit content of the right brain of the two members of the therapeutic couple and its own way of being. With F.R. the time of despair and tormenting feelings without form lasted two years: "Only to you can I say these things … the others would take me for a fool … I fear I am a fool …." In each session he would ask me if I understood his complaints and if I remembered what he had told me over time. He had a constant need to be reminded as if it was up to me to hold him together, as in him the perception of internal experience was divided into distinct emotions and "atomised debris" (Ferenczi, 2017). A full perception of self was absent. He was afraid of this and feared that this lack of internal coherence could lead him to madness and the possibility of suicide. He always had to make sure that I did not feel confused; thus, in every session of the first period, he repeatedly asked me if I understood what he had told me while he was despairing and crying. In fact, it was not easy to understand his fragmented speeches and complaints. They were jumbled fragments of complaints. Every rare attempt at interpretation was angrily rejected because he feared I would drive him even crazier with those speeches.

Thus, gradually my listening began to take on the pattern of a fluctuating attention, marked by moments of empathic contact and a tolerance to stand in a vacuum, in an indistinct immersion in his complaints. A participatory and at the same time distracted listening, during a timeless time, where emotions did not take shape, but only expressed themselves with the sound of his complaints. As I listened, I no longer tried to trace them back to some rational form.

The sessions were thus characterised for a couple of years by my long silences, dedicated to listening, and the assertion that he was not crazy, but suffered from a personality disorder. It was not appropriate for me to add any clarification, he would angrily rebel. In essence, he asked me for a total and primitive listening, as in a relationship that, having regressed from the Oedipal events, had become stranded in a defective dyadic relationship, laden with hyper-emotional sensoriality. What was needed at that time was a kind of deep, instinctive acceptance on my part. I had to perform the function of offering a calming and ordering rhythm, waiting for the right time to create representations where they were lacking. I recalled Giovanni Hautmann's considerations expressed in seminars at the AFPP on the primitive role of visual experience which, anticipating spoken experience, constituted a kind of immediate mutual recognition. Thus, the first act of the session consisted of a lengthy mutual observation from the moment the door was opened and a repetition of this ritual at the moment of leave-taking, as if attempting to maintain the imprint of what was emotionally experienced. Sessions in which from beginning to end he despaired about his tormenting feelings while I repeated that it was only the result of anxiety, filled a long time.

Then a type of evolution took place and a certain sense of progressive, smiling good-natured humour was naturally introduced into our relationship, in welcoming me in his aggressive attacks and him in teasing me in my authoritarian firmness. A somewhat irreverent game in which we joked about each other's character traits; almost like a gentle caress that had the sense of a more intimate recognition, increasingly coloured by affectionate intonations.

At a later stage, when the complaints had become rarer, the time finally came when I proposed that the patient engage in constructive experiences, in contrast to the neutral psychoanalytic technical abstinence. Every now and then he made sure I did not forget what he had told me, as if my reply, which punctually arrived, had the function of banishing the thought that he counted for nothing for me. I would respond, deliberately, after a few sessions, in a seemingly casual manner, recalling some episode he had mentioned many sessions before.

After two years, the patient and his partner began the long, interminable journey of artificial insemination during which he remained constantly at her side, while I was invested with the role of witnessing the anxiety evoked by the events of a complicated pregnancy. At the same time, F.R., with his partner, had arranged a room for their daughter, who was born at the beginning of 2021, and who "by chance" was given the same name that I had given my daughter 30 years ago...

Notes

1 The fundamental characteristics identified by Kernberg consisted of non-specific manifestations of ego weakness, such as difficulty tolerating anxiety; deficits in impulse control; absence of mature sublimatory modalities; ease of primary thought processes; primitive defences and non-integrated good/bad object relations.
2 Compromising self-identity; anaclitic relationships; depression linked to a sense of isolation and predominance of expressed anger.
3 The structures involved (Hart, 2008) consist of the cingulate gyrus, which induces attachment-related emotional behaviour; the parietal lobe, which maintains a sense of internal subjective space; the insula, which integrates representations of somatic states; and the orbitofrontal cortex, which connects imaginary stimuli with emotional reactions, coordinating emotional manifestations with thoughts to make mentalisation possible, and managing them appropriately.

References

Adler, G. (1985). *Borderline Psychopathology and Its Treatment.* New York: Jason Aronson.

Bateman, A., Fonagy, P. and Allen, J.G. (2009). Theory and Practice of Mentalization-Based Therapy. In G.O. Gabbard (ed.), *Textbook of Psychotherapeutic Treatments.* Washington, DC: American Psychiatric Publishing, pp. 757–780. Available at: psycnet.apa.org.

Battle, C.L. *et al.* (2004). Childhood Maltreatment Associated with Adult Personality Disorders: Findings from the Collaborative Longitudinal Personality Disorders Study. *Journal of Personality Disorders,* 4: 193–211.

Beebe, B. and Lachmann, F. (2002). Organizing Principles of Interaction from Infant Research and the Lifespan Prediction of Attachment: Application to Adult Treatment. *Journal of Infant, Child and Adolescent Psychotherapy,* 2: 61–89.

Beebe, B. and Lachmann, F. (2003). The Relational Turn in Psychoanalysis: A Dyadic Systems View from Infant Research. *Contemporary Psychoanalysis,* 39: 379–409.

Beebe, B., Lachmann, F. and Jaffe, J. (1997). Mother-Infant Structures and Presymbolic Self and Object Representation. *Psychoanalytic Dialogues,* 7: 133–182.

Bolognini, S. (2008). *Passaggi segreti: teoria e tecnica della relazione interpsichica.* Turin: Bollati Boringhieri.

De Masi, F. (2013). Borderline: un paziente senza inconscio? Available at: SPIWeb (accessed 17 January 2013).

Ferenczi, S. (2017). *The Clinical Diary (January–October 1932).* London: Routledge.

Grinker, R. (1968). *The Borderline Syndrome: A Behavioural Study of Ego Functions.* London: Basic Books.

Gunderson, J. and Ridolfi, M. (2001). Borderline Personality Disorder: Suicidality and Self-Mutilation. *Annals of the New York Academy of Sciences,* 932: 60–83.

Hart, S. (2008). *Brain, Attachment, Personality.* London: Karnac.

Kernberg, O. (1967). Borderline Personality Organization. *Journal of the American Psychoanalytic Association,* 15: 641–685.

Kernberg, O. (1975). *Borderline Conditions and Pathological Narcissism.* New York: Jason Aronson.

Knight, R.P. (1953). Management and Psychotherapy of the Borderline Schizophrenic Patient. *Bulletin of the Menninger Clinic,* 17: 139–150.

Knight, R.P. (1954). Borderline States. In R.P. Knight and C.R. Friedman (eds), *Psychoanalytic Psychiatry and Psychology*. New York: International Universities Press, pp. 97–109.

Mancia, M. (1994). *Dall'Edipo al sogno. Modelli della mente nello sviluppo e nel transfert*. Milan: Raffaello Cortina.

Mancia, M. (2003). Implicit Memory and Unrepressed Unconscious: Their Role in Creativity and Transference. *Israel Psychoanalytic Journal*, 3: 331–349.

Ponsi, M. (2012a). Evoluzione del pensiero psicoanalitico. Acting out, agire, enactment. *Rivista di Psicoanalisi*, 58: 653–670.

Ponsi, M. (2012b). L'enactment nel processo analitico. Commento alla relazione di A. Schore "Un cambiamento di paradigma nell'approccio terapeutico agli enactments". Interview with Allan Shore, Rome, October 20–21, 2012. Available at: SPIWeb (accessed 19 June 2013).

Shore, A.N. (2003). *Affect Dysregulation and Disorders of the Self*. New York: W.W. Norton & Company.

Shore, A.N. (2012). *The Science of the Art of Psychotherapy*. New York: W.W. Norton & Company.

Spitzer, R. and Endicott, J. (1979). Justification for Separating Schizotypal and Borderline Personality Disorders. *Schizophrenia Bulletin*, 5: 95–104.

Stern, A. (1938). Psychoanalytic Investigation of and Therapy in the Borderline Group of Neuroses. *Psychoanalytic Quarterly*, 7: 467–489.

Chapter 8

Psychotherapy and artistic expression

Cristina D. Canzio

Exploring the relationship between psychoanalytic psychotherapy and artistic expression has always raised questions that I believe must be answered. Can we consider psychotherapy to be related to artistic expression? What do they have in common? Is psychotherapy an art? If so, what kind of art is it? In which aspects can these two identities resemble each other? Does something creative reside in that "space-journey" that patient and therapist build together? Therefore, I would like to start by expressing some ideas about creativity and its function in the life experience of every individual.

To be creative, a person must exist and feel that they exist not only consciously but as the basis of their own actions. Creativity is something that emerges within the individual when there is an element of "doing" involved, giving their "feeling" a sense of being alive.

The impulse to "do" may sometimes seem dormant, but when it emerges, creativity appears. It is necessary for an activity that constitutes a strong motivation to "move" and engage in constructive action, to prevail over an activity that is purely reactive and would result in a behavior "void of meaning."

The question of creativity processes is significant in psychoanalysis because it also concerns what takes place between the therapist and the patient in the transference and countertransference relationship. We know that transference can no longer be considered merely acceptance or resignation, and that it is also subject to limitations. If transference unfolds in a transitional area within the unintegrated part of the ego, allowing creativity to unfold beyond symbolization, then it certainly becomes richer, evolves, and expands.

In his (1971) essay, "Creativity and its Origins," Winnicott begins with the following wish:

> I hope the reader will accept a general reference to creativity without allowing the word to be lost and confused with successful or acclaimed creation, but instead keep it limited to the meaning that refers to a kind of coloring of the internal attitude towards external reality.

DOI: 10.4324/9781032673721-9

The orientation established during the process of emotional maturation and the factors that influence it the most are those that are implemented from the beginning of existence. And that is precisely how we can think of creativity: as something that belongs fully to the infantile experience but can last a lifetime, preserving and prolonging the ability to create the world, "our" world.

As we know, the reality principle belongs to the very existence of the world, regardless of whether the child believes in it or not. In sufficiently good environmental conditions, the child can find various ways to assimilate the events they have experienced, thanks to their own resources of "creativity." They can form their own opinion about everything.

Through a complex process of genetically determined maturation, combined with interactions between individual maturation and environmental factors that can be either facilitating or maladaptive and inducing reactions, the child who has grown into an adult has acquired the ability to see things in a new way, to "be creative" in every aspect of their existence. Creativity associated with the sensation of being alive helps the child in their growth process to relate to objects, guiding and supporting them in their efforts to fulfill their desires and needs.

The laws of the universe offer everyone the possibility to live creatively. This means preserving something personal – who knows, a secret – that is unequivocally one's own.

When we live creatively, we discover that everything we do strengthens our sense of self-esteem and being ourselves. Of course, we are talking about living a creative life, feeling alive, not artistic creation where a person is expected to showcase some talent. To live creatively, one does not need any special talent; it is both a universal necessity and a universal experience.

We are all aware of the value of the transitional space, where the emotional dimension develops and the construction of the sense of existence takes place, regardless of the presence or absence of others – that feeling of being loved, being involved in a relationship, not being exposed to the unknown, even though we well know how important and necessary it is to learn to tolerate the unknown.

It is therefore a space that holds a relationship, witnessing the exclusively shared emotional dimension with the parent/therapist. It is also a tool that takes shape through interaction and can be used to symbolically relive all the emotions associated with the presence of the other, thus fostering the development of a true self, where the creativity of the individual finds an adequate space for expression.

According to Winnicott, one of the necessary aspects for the development of a true self is the capacity to be alone, in the absence or presence of others. The ability to be alone is also the ability to be oneself without having to please others. This can only be achieved through early experiences or in the therapeutic experience in adulthood.

As we know, play allows the child to see things from the external world invested with new meaning: a piece of wood becomes a horse that the child happily gallops on, and even scribbles become a way of playing and communicating. Play represents the birth of creative thought. Initially, it is expressed through the bond the child has with the mother, and later it evolves into the ability to turn objects into symbols, transforming matter into a "spiritual" reality that accompanies the individual.

A fundamental characteristic of human beings is the ability to give meaning to what they do and the objects they produce. With the production of transitional objects, the mind demonstrates its ability to create symbolic objects, enabling the development of arts, religion, imaginative life, and scientific creation.

Although art does not have a therapeutic purpose, it has the potential to show us and make us reflect on certain unconscious psychic dynamics and mechanisms. Our ghosts, our imagination, are projected onto the text or the canvas, resonating with the depicted or painted subject that the artist – or the one who draws or writes – captures in its essence. In psychotherapy, they emerge as a result of the work woven between patient and therapist. In this model, a representation comes to represent an "intermediate area of experience" between the self and the external world.

I also refer to the "consideration" of the therapist's creativity in its desirable moments, particularly in their daily clinical work with patients, where creativity is comparable to that of an artist at work. This is the artistic-creative dimension of psychotherapy as a profession.

Beyond the transitional device

The purpose of creating a transitional device is to support the individual, allowing new ideas to emerge – including fantasies and attempts to create a good enough environment that enables "invention." This requires the therapist to engage in listening as a connection and openness to understanding the patient's suffering, obstacles, and difficulties, while simultaneously creating conditions that allow for expression, action, and play, even in dialogue.

In psychotherapy, the aim is often to "play what has never been played before." Thus, in a "listening game," where there is always total respect for the other, for what is "unique" about the other, with their personal and specific rhythms, beliefs, and limitations, a movement, a fluidity of all those transitions that have remained stagnant and imprisoned can be restored. These transitions make themselves heard by the therapist through the discomfort experienced when listening to certain unresolved materials.

"To think while playing," that is, to find a way to transition from passivity to a state of activity, including the suffering of an unspeakable reality, in order to construct a "fiction" that allows for the processing of a piece of one's own experiences: this encounter between patient and therapist – which is outside of time but within a bond – is what should promote the free ability to be "used" by the patient in a new territory of the internal-external that flows, transfers, and transforms into an intermediate space. In this way, the therapist's listening becomes a connection that facilitates the creation of conditions to thaw the stagnant development.

Winnicott took play seriously, rediscovering it as a simultaneously destructive and creative expression. Becoming is a category that invites us to think beyond the logic of beginning and end, that is, to depart from one place to arrive at another. In becoming, things are caught halfway, they are those spaces where processes occur, the space that exists and flows between two limits. Becoming and the transitional space are paradoxical categories because they do not refer to time but rather to space. However, they do refer to a founding space of time, offering the possibility of initiating a process.

The concept of microanalysis, as proposed by E. Smalinsky (2021). invites us to think not of the grand classical psychoanalysis that has a beginning and an end, but rather of small microanalyses conducted over time. We can think of psychoanalytic psychotherapy more as an opportunity to be present, without aiming to create a beginning or an end, without concern for being, and seeking to restore the patient's ability to play, speak, and express themselves as they please, where the therapist allows them to encounter that intermediate zone of experience.

Psychic suffering can arise whenever the failure to create oneself, the impossibility of organizing aesthetic conflict, and initiating the process of subjectivity become apparent. Therapeutic work, then, consists of generating the conditions for the processing of those aspects – often invisible and often silent – experienced in sustaining the transference.

In the classical perspective of psychoanalysis, listening is privileged with the aim of promoting the process of making the unconscious conscious. However, any therapist working with more or less severe patients or children will have realized that literal listening is not entirely adequate for effective therapy. When Freud conceived the analytic process as a mode of symbolization, comparing that process to children's play as another way of symbolizing, he did not grasp the importance of the differences between the two processes and considered free association as equivalent to play.

Later, Melanie Klein introduced play into the treatment of children, supported by playing with the therapist, thus initiating the development of Kleinian thought, which considers art as reparation, while Freud believed that cultural objects expressed, evoked, and represented the outcome of internal themes and conflicts, emphasizing the continuity between art and other modes of mental functioning, such as wit and dreams.

Freud writes in "The Poet and Fantasy" (1907 [1989]): "Perhaps it can be said that every child engaged in play behaves like a poet: as they construct their own world or, rather, give to their pleasure a new arrangement of things in their world." This outlines the image of a child artist who rearranges objects in strange configurations according to their taste and pleasure, thus paving the way for Winnicott.

Therefore, it is not about making the unconscious conscious, as Freud said, but rather about making a "passage," realizing the minimal transitions necessary to maintain the existence of an intermediate area that allows for the articulation of the internal and external worlds, avoiding blind adaptation to the environment. The clinical work with severely disturbed patients and children shows that the ability to speak and play develops throughout the therapeutic process, aided by the introduction of elements that assist the patient in expressing themselves differently, facilitating symbolization and deeper, more fruitful communication.

Fernando Ulloa (2012) argued that a "deadly pact" must be made, meaning that for suffering to become accessible for symbolization, both the patient and the therapist need to find a way to move beyond the passivity and submission they experience in response to certain contents expressed in the therapeutic relationship. In this regard, the transitional space (which allows for an active position) seems useful as a pathway to reach symbolization.

The clinical case I present here illustrates a bridge through which to access mental pathways, usually unconscious, capable of leading to inner transformation, whereby feelings, emotions, and fragmented pieces of painful experiences acquire meaning and significance through their representation.

The introduction of a blank sheet can serve as a silent support onto which colors are placed, where the starting point of watercolor becomes a challenge, a risk, but also a discreet, reserved, and absent support for various chromatic shades, attempting to give form to silence and underpin words to express themselves.

The patient – whom I will call Anna – is a 34-year-old woman who has been undergoing psychotherapy on a weekly basis for a year and a half. The reason that led her to embark on a journey of self-discovery is the desire to understand what drives her to explode with arguments and disputes when something doesn't go her way, with a feeling of rejection and abandonment.

After a year of therapy, the young woman brings a painting to the session (Figure 8.1). commenting that she made it to represent an inner part of herself that feels darker and imprisoned, causing her great suffering because she can't express it in her relationships with others.

She explains that she decided to create this painting using black and burgundy colors to represent that inner part of herself that she has tried to silence for years but somehow it always manages to surface and make itself heard.

She tells me that while painting, she needed to explain to herself what she was experiencing during that period, getting to know her own shadows without judgment, allowing them to speak through the images that emerged in her mind. "And here," she says, "in that dark room, a small window opens at the top." She continues, "Because without darkness, there would be no light."

"Thus, I understood," she adds, "that the light has always been there inside me, among the extinguished lights of the room that inhabit my soul. For me, each room represents something that marked me in the past and somehow

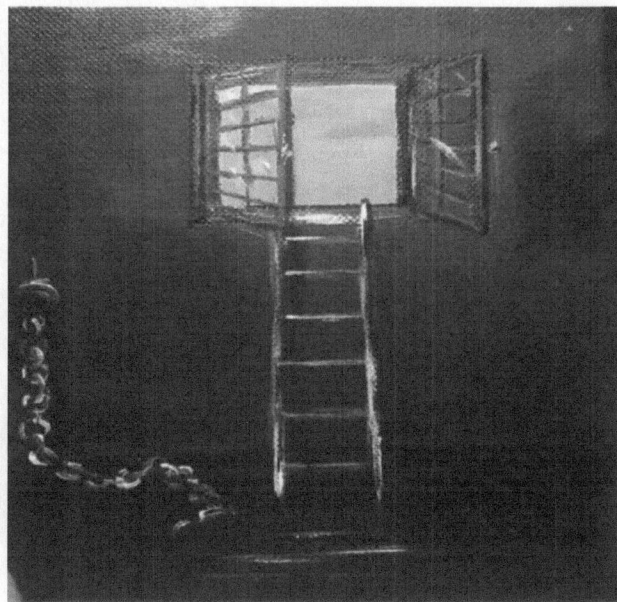

Figure 8.1 From darkness to light

influences my daily choices. But when I think that in every room, there is a window through which light enters, I remember that I can face my fears and confront them. This gives me a sense of reality that makes me believe I am always the one who can choose. I added the chain afterwards: a more descriptive detail because I feared that anyone looking at the painting wouldn't be able to understand the concept of what I wanted to represent."

Later on, she brought me another painting (Figure 8.2).

She explained: "When I started this painting, I didn't have a clear idea of what I wanted to represent, but I knew I wanted light. So, I painted a sky with marvelous shades, reminiscent of the beautiful walks among the Tuscan hills and the nature of summer. The past two summers have been exciting and filled with gratitude for me: during the first one, I walked the Via Francigena and felt life flowing through my veins. The sun warmed my face and my heart. I will never forget those sensations. But even stronger was the experience of the following summer in Val d'Orcia with my boyfriend. And that's when my painting transformed into a gentle ascent, framed by the beauty of nature, beyond which you can almost touch the sky with a fingertip and imagine a breathtaking panorama."

These two drawings have helped confirm my intuition regarding your "willingness to know" – in a Bionian sense – where you are able to convey a feeling, an experience that is important beyond words. The patient allows us to enter an unknown part of herself, where we can visualize her internal

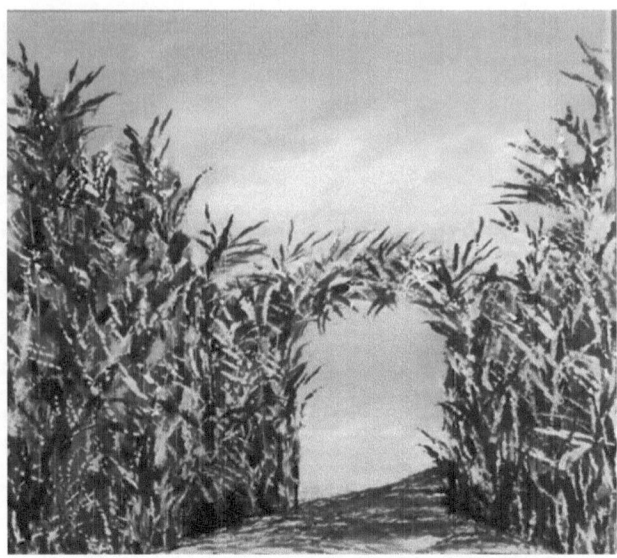

Figure 8.2 Nature in summertime

process and how she navigates it to symbolize her own emotional state. Through her narrative, we can appreciate her ability to formulate thoughts and represent them as a sign of containment.

This new acquisition of emotional containment (sometimes fluctuating) is supported by the therapist's capacity for "reverie," leading the patient to expand her ability to tolerate frustration by reliving it through her mode of representation, rather than avoiding or evacuating it as bad and painful content, as she previously did with aggressive reactions, provocative responses, anger outbursts, and abandoning relationships with others (which is why she sought treatment).

The transformation the patient undergoes can be observed in this second drawing, with a luminous green arch and an uphill road leading to an open space like a clear sky, capable of conveying to the observer a desire for joy, clarity, and the search for serenity.

The patient brings this painting with great apprehension but eagerly awaits my opinion. I receive it with curiosity and satisfaction, and as both of us gaze upon the painted image, we feel that something has changed, a sky opens up before our observing eyes, something has happened, something has been altered, the evidence is right there before our eyes.

This well-represented inner image gives rise to its creative output. We can paraphrase Bion (1962) by saying, "the apparatus for thinking thoughts is under construction." A path has been opened to process the anxiety of separation by choosing one's own freedom of expression.

In psychoanalytic psychotherapy, we speak of the possibility of construct-ing a valid container through a strong bond of therapeutic love that conveys presence, empathy, and willingness to listen to emotions during the ther-apeutic relationship. "The patient – and only the patient – knows what it feels like to be oneself," Bion reminds us.

The patient sent me this latest painting via WhatsApp, as due to the pan-demic, we were conducting remote sessions (Figure 8.3).

Here, she wanted to represent the four seasons, their circular repetition, where one season ends while the other begins, a circle just like life. "The trunk of the tree is me," she says, "with a fixed root in the ground while the seasons of life change, the leaves on the branches: there are the fragrant ones that are life, and the others that fall are death."

"Water has two meanings," she says. "Water is life because we are made of water. But it is also death, metaphorical death because in it, we can reflect on ourselves when we mirror ourselves in the water, losing everything that happens around us, as if time stopped."

"I associate this death with narcissism," she continues, referring to Caravaggio's painting, saying, "because to enjoy my image, I am not interested in anything else. The mountains with the little woods indicate an unknown depth full of cold, gloomy, while next to them, there are the hills that convey peace and freedom to me. In the end, the four seasons are not delimited by a boundary line because I don't believe that the transition from one season to another in life is so abrupt but rather gradual, like a shade." Here we see how Anna's ghosts and imagination

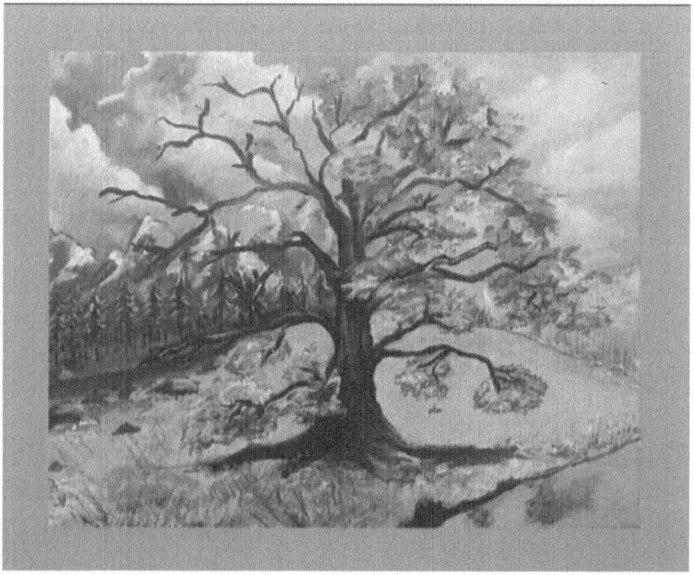

Figure 8.3 The four seasons

project onto the painting due to some resonances with what has been depicted and what she tells with great ease.

We know that the great machine that transforms the experience of the internal world into thought is mourning. Loss sets in motion processes that create thoughts, and Anna's creativity paves the way for the search for the lost object, which then appears in her drawings as something new that will never be the original object but a condensation of many intertwined and scattered materials.

This demonstrates the capacity and internal organization with which a skilled human being can draw from their internal processes (libido) to change a destiny marked by traumatic childhood situations, trying to escape from them. The patient expresses the possibility of self-understanding, construction, and renewal, thus confirming that the ego must follow a necessary path to reach sublimated form and abstraction. This growth process consists of processing the loss.

These identifications, which fundamentally underlie the psychic structure, confirm the fact that we are "constructed" by others, but it will depend on the manner and mode in which these others organize and reorganize themselves through the processing of the "lost object" during the therapeutic process and how one can become someone in particular by constructing their own uniqueness.

As Gabbard (2010) reminds us, it is necessary to find a space where therapist and patient can communicate effectively. Finding this space can be an important challenge in treatment. The patient sent this latest painting recently with the inscription: "I think hands are an extension of the mind" (Figure 8.4).

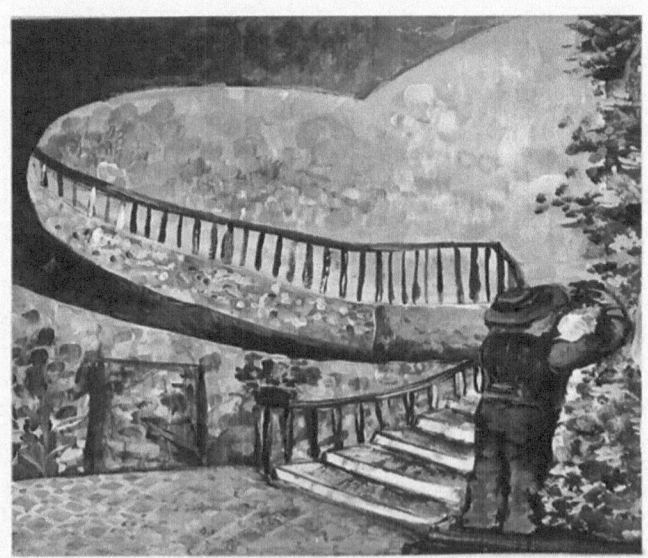

Figure 8.4 Taking care by hands end by mind

I want to conclude by quoting from Marcel Proust (1990), cited in Monniello (2018), which pertains to the actual creation of oneself:

> It is known that in certain afflictions of the nervous system, the patient, without any particular organ being affected, is trapped in a sort of inability to will, as if in a deep ditch from which they cannot escape on their own, and where they would wither away if a powerful and helpful hand did not reach out to them.
>
> There are some spirits comparable to these patients, whom a sort of laziness or frivolity prevents from spontaneously descending into the deep regions of themselves where the true life of the spirit begins. Once led there, they are capable of discovering and exploiting its true riches, but without this external intervention, they live on the surface in a perpetual forgetfulness of themselves, in a kind of passivity that makes them prey to all pleasures … They would eventually erase any memory of their spiritual nobility if an external impulse did not bring them back, somehow forcing them, to the life of the spirit, where they suddenly regain the power to think for themselves and create.

References

Bion, W.R. (1962). *Learning from Experience*. London: Routledge.

Freud, S. (1908 [1989]). Il poeta e la fantasia. In *OSF*, vol. 5. Turin: Bollati Boringhieri.

Gabbard, G.O. (2010). *Long-Term Psychodynamic Psychotherapy*. Washington, DC: American Psychiatric Publishing.

Monniello, G. (2018). La Psicoanalisi tra le arti. Available at: https://www.spiweb.it/wp content/uploads/oldfiles/images/stories/psicoana-lisi e arte fertile incontro.pdf (accessed 15 February 2022).

Proust, M. (1990). *A la recherche du temps perdu*, vol. 7: *Le Temps retrouvé*. Paris: Edition Gallimard.

Smalinsky, E. (2021). *Devenir jugando*. Buenos Aires: Edition Brueghel.

Ulloa, F. (2012). *Novela psicoanalitica*. Buenos Aires: Libros El Zorzal.

Winnicott, D.W. (1971). Creativity and its Origins. In *Playing and Reality*. London: Tavistock Publications.

Chapter 9

"Leading our caravans to the West"[1]

Psychotherapy at a distance

Cristina Pratesi

Talking about psychoanalytic psychotherapy today would not be complete if we did not also refer to what happened in our professional practice due to the COVID-19 pandemic.

The use of online therapy is certainly nothing new: as early as 2003, P. Migone (2003) wrote on psychoanalysis and online psychotherapy, also mentioning the practice of telephone analysis that began in the United States in the mid-1900s (Saul, 1951), ascribing it to the broader chapter of telemedicine, which had been experimented with for years, especially over very large geographical areas, where distances were in fact sometimes an insurmountable obstacle, not least because of costs.

In Italy, too, we know how online consultations, such as the use of chats in listening and help services for juvenile distress, especially peer-to-peer for adolescents and their families[2] with the external support of a psychotherapist, and the use of programs and platforms for real-time video calls (Skype, Zoom, Jitsi, Meet, for instance) have taken off over the years.

The outbreak of the Coronavirus emergency and the consequent lockdown have, however, forced an acceleration towards the use of online tools, given the impossibility of maintaining the classic set-ups of the sessions.[3] As A.M. Nicolò (2020) reminds us, online analysis represents a real revolution because it forces us to rethink and readjust all the parameters and all those aspects that we have so far indicated as fundamental in the construction of the therapeutic container, which leads us to ask ourselves "whether the results we can achieve are comparable to in-person work and whether, despite so many drastic differences, work on the unconscious remains possible". Let us consider, for example, some peculiarities of working via Skype and video or telephone call. The real body is missing: that of the patient, but also that of the therapist. The image is mediated by a screen or even absent, the perceptions are missing, as well as the sensory contact between patient and therapist, with all those "multiple, subtle body channels" we spoke about earlier. Even the "musical listening" of verbal and non-verbal sound messages is somewhat limited, as is the possibility of speaking actions and "InterpretActions".

DOI: 10.4324/9781032673721-10

There are no longer concretely "two people talking in a room" (Nissim Momigliano, 1984), but there is a new space (cyberspace[4]) in which, however, the task and function of the therapist remain stable, and he/she must be – now more than ever – able and willing to reach out to the patient "wherever he or she may be, shedding his or her own clothes and putting himself or herself on the other's side ... the dialogue that one sees developing between patient and analyst resembles a four-hands sonata".

Listening seems to consist – again, more than ever – in paying attention to what is happening at that moment "between" patient and psychotherapist, "often giving up interpreting what is happening in the patient" (Nissim Momigliano, 1984).

Paraphrasing the definition that A. Robutti (2001) coined for L. Nissim Momigliano, we find ourselves having to be psychotherapists "capable of change".

What we have to deal with is no small matter:

- Only the upper part of the patient's and the therapist's body is visible, which inevitably brings our thoughts back to what D. Meltzer theorised (Fano Cassese, 2001) regarding the split that some patients operate unconsciously in their internal world: a horizontal split that divides an upper part of the body (the face and breasts), which is experienced as beautiful, good, nourishing, and a lower part, a place of aspects to be hidden, bad and dirty. It seems important to me to bear in mind how in some situations the screen, which shows only the upper part of the body can actually function as a reinforcement of the defensive denial of these parts.[5]
- Even if one looks directly at the screen, the other person will not be looked in the eye – which would only happen by staring at the webcam and thus effectively giving up seeing the other person's face.
- We enter an "elsewhere" different from the usual setting: we access, albeit invited, the patient's private space, we see his or her living or working environment. Those of us who have worked with terminally ill patients in palliative care services know well how, in some cases, working at home enriches rather than hinders the psychotherapist's perspective. Especially when time is necessarily and forcibly short, entering the patient's home allows and facilitates getting closer to his or her internal world. As A. Eiguer states:

"The home is a reflection of who we are ... it is a functioning model where the human reproduces what he lives within himself ... it is a psychic representation, a synthesis of the representation of his own body and that of the family group ... the home represents a very delicate theme, being pervaded by emotion, nostalgia, history".

(2004)

Moreover, it is not always possible for the therapist to connect while remaining in his or her office, so he or she will operate a kind of self-disclosure, while trying to keep as anonymous and neutral as possible the portion of space that the patient can see from the screen, in order to ensure a proper therapeutic process and to protect the projective transference dynamics.

- Cyberpsychology researchers, who are studying the effects of the use of this type of tool and online work more generally, point to the emergence of the phenomenon of so-called "zoom fatigue", a feeling of excessive mental exhaustion, from which as psychotherapists we are not immune. The sense of increased fatigue, as if to "pierce the screen" and reach the patient empathically, is reported by many of us, who sometimes also have to deal with technological failures: poor connections, poor image quality and non-synchronisation between audio and video.
- It is common for the therapist to report finding himself looking at himself, at his own image, also present in a small way on the screen, that is, almost as a participant observer/spectator of what the patient sees (I observe my own image, which reaches the patient and which the patient sees). The gaze, therefore, no longer seems to play the role of a "visual container" but opens up to a game of cross-references and mirroring.
- All the more so in telephone sessions, apart from the "absence of body contact" (Suman, 2022), the function of the gaze does not exist. In a telephone session, the whole set of sensations is almost non-existent in favour of an increased perception of rhythm, breath, hesitations and stumbles of the voice, semi-lapses and repetitions of words. Our interlocutor searches for the therapist who is silent, restless, imagining a broken communication (Richard, 2020).

Silences, an important part of classical sessions, here can activate anxiety, bewilderment, feelings comparable to a "horror vacui" especially at a time like the pandemic when there is danger lurking outside, a devious threat, and already the anxiety of death pervades everything and everyone. It is the voice that is the only link, the only connection, the only security, which reminds us of Freud (1905 [2001]): "Aunt, speak to me, I am afraid of the dark." The aunt then answered him: "But what's the use? You don't see me anyway." "It doesn't matter," the child retorted, "if someone talks, there is light." Working at a distance, via telephone, can therefore certainly constitute a supportive, anxiety-reducing aspect, but something else takes place as well:

> in psychotherapy sessions by telephone, as in *Solo Piano* concerts, the use of *Solo Voice*, in the absence of other stimuli … can be for some less distracting and uncover a *Tone* that is usually outclassed by the evocative power of the perception of other elements.
>
> (Lisciotto, 2020)

It can also facilitate the disclosure of otherwise censored and embarrassing memories: "I don't know why I had never told her about this episode before.

Maybe I'm less ashamed on the phone?" says M., 40, after one year of therapy, recalling an episode when, he as a teenager, sexually harassed a little cousin.

These "makeshift settings" that we were forced to set up in no time at all, on the basis of the emergency (Bolognini, 2020), allowed us not to suspend the sessions, thus leaving the patient in an indefinite temporal dimension full of anxious uncertainties (dissimilar from holiday separations, where the date of return is defined); instead, they sometimes illuminated – like a spotlight on the stage – aspects relating to areas that are otherwise split off or inhibited, transgressive or which have remained until then in the background. The following cases are explanatory in this regard.

Clinical cases

Case X[6]

Mr. X. is 50 years old and has been in weekly one-to-one, face-to-face therapy for about a year following the separation from his wife. He has a harmless good-guy appearance, a responsible job in which he is respected by superiors and colleagues, constantly practises sports to keep fit and is very religious, bordering on bigotry. Although he has no concrete proof, he is convinced that he has been betrayed by his wife since the early years of their marriage and reports bloody fantasies of revenge, resulting in uxoricide and the murder of his rival. For years, he was subject to frequent fits of rage, during which he verbally attacked and humiliated his partner, who eventually asked for and obtained a divorce, despite her outright opposition on religious grounds. In therapy, he behaves like a good boy and explains why he resists the strong desire to carry out revenge, referring in a very childish and egocentric way to religious dictates ("You can't do it because it is a mortal sin and I would end up in hell"). For the Coronavirus emergency, the sessions have to forcibly shift to Skype, which the patient uses on a tablet, sitting on a couch in his home. The therapist begins to feel very different sensations from those experienced during the sessions in the office, physical sensations, such as seasickness and nausea: the patient never holds the tablet still and therefore the image on the screen is not only in a continuous, paroxysmal movement, but the therapist almost never manages to see the patient, who frames instead the ceiling of the room or at most the top of his head, i.e., the hair and the forehead, only sometimes the eyes. Subsequently, in addition to seasickness, the therapist begins to experience sensations of extreme disgust, with respect to parts of the body which the patient casually and fleetingly frames in his perpetual motion of the tablet: for example, the part of an arm, uncovered because the patient is wearing a half-sleeved shirt, which the therapist perceives as "whitish, flabby and repulsive". Or the nose, which is framed as the patient is picking his nose, something never done during the sessions. In contrast, the therapist realises that she takes on a very rigid posture and impassive expression, just as the patient speaks of his ex-wife, describing her as "stiff and impenetrable".

Case Y[7]

Y. started psychotherapy at the age of 18, following the advice of his psychiatrist, after an emergency admission in a psychiatric unit, where he was diagnosed with a brief psychotic disorder.

After about two years of one-week face-to-face psychotherapy, characterised, however, by two long intervals,[8] Y. moved abroad and the sessions took place via Skype. The therapist notes:

> The introduction of Skype was certainly a critical issue, it was a novelty that required an adaptation of our way of being together and even today there are moments when we both struggle a lot in front of the screen … while waiting for this new meeting, I admit that I did not prepare myself much for using Skype. Realizing the great change taking place with the passage from a real meeting to a virtual one, I preferred to proceed inductively, starting from what was going to happen and letting myself be guided, at least not at first, by the facts … I therefore tried to think of the path via Skype as a 'change of clothes' and not something totally and fearfully new (Ferro, 2013). I am very excited about this new 'departure' and imagine the meeting with Y. as a moment full of stories and emotions. But reality turns out to be quite different from this fantasy of mine and the first session is very difficult and at times incomprehensible. Among my notes from the session I find these words:
>
> > *We know each other but we cannot recognize each other. Seeing each other through the screen, after years of face-to-face therapy and after more than three months of interruption, makes us awkward. I immediately realise the criticality of the transition from real to virtual encounters. I feel something is missing and I find myself displaced. I miss the greeting at the door, I miss noticing his posture, I miss walking down the corridor to the room with him, the gestures, the small movements, the smells… I miss all those elements that go beyond words but which often allow us to feel, imagine and understand. After the first few minutes I feel my initial enthusiasm inappropriate and I have to scale back my excitement. I feel there is a wall and an emptiness.*

This initial difficulty is followed by a period which the therapist describes as:

> like a seascape after a big storm. We have to sit down, look at it together and get used to the changes … Y. seems to live a life that is not his own,

he does not realise what is happening and I perceive a constant avoidant tendency, as a defence mechanism against anxious thinking … there is a marked tendency to evacuate thoughts and contents in an almost aggressive way, never used before in a session … Y. and his companion's house becomes a kind of sea-port, where various people come and go: his companion's sister, Y.'s father, mother and brother. The house is always crowded and Y. lives at the mercy of events, in the midst of turmoil, deeply disoriented. He cannot carve out a space of his own, he shows me this difficulty and makes me realise that he does not feel looked at and respected by anyone. Therapy, in fact, suffers from all this chaos … these presences crowd the patient's mind and even our space: on a couple of occasions I was forced to interrupt the session because his partner or other relatives were walking behind Y. while he was trying to talk to me. I believe that the use of Skype with the camera pointed inside the walls of his house facilitated the communication of the very strong chaos experienced by my patient during this period: virtual reality helped a lot by showing the harshness of everyday reality. In all this chaos and the comings and goings of people, the thing that left me dismayed was the apparent total unawareness of the inappropriateness of certain situations for the purposes of our work … I started to rethink about Y. and us. Certainly the change of setting after the first two years from face-to-face to Skype was an element that destabilised us, making the meeting new and more difficult: on the one hand, Skype distanced us from our bodies and this represented an important and significant novelty as it allowed us to limit the invasion of corporeity (which was a very important element during therapy); on the other hand, it is as if Skype and the video calls had, in fact, distanced and shielded even the emotions and their expression … a very pregnant image emerged to describe the patient's use of the sessions before and after Skype: for Y. face-to-face therapy was a warm place/object, a warm, welcoming place/object, for Y. a warm, welcoming and nourishing place/object, a "breast" with which he could feel, grow and support himself; the use of Skype led him to use the sessions not so much as a nourishing object but as a sort of "dummy", a consoling, calming, but at times masturbatory surrogate.

In both cases reported, the use of Skype allowed the therapist: on the one hand, to concretely see and experience situations that the patient was experiencing, but of which he was not yet fully aware (i.e., the resonance that the external world had in his internal world and vice versa); on the other hand, to grasp, through his countertransference, fundamental aspects of the patient's psychopathology that had remained in the shadows. All this is particularly true with regard to those psychotherapies that began in the studio, with the classic working modalities, and that for different reasons, as it was with the COVID-19 lockdown, had to "transmigrate" online. Be that as it may, even in a modified, apparently distorted setting, the patient continues to bring his own internal world into the session: it is therefore up to the therapist to keep his own internal psychic set-up solid and authentic, in order to "create an analysing situation despite, with, a priori, a state of affairs that does not lend itself well to it" (Richard, 2020).

Back East

While there have been indeed many scientific contributions aimed at promoting a common reflection on the impact of the pandemic and its lockdown on psychoanalytic psychotherapy practice, also examining what was going on in the minds of we therapists, the resonances provoked in our internal world, as well as in the external one, by the changes in professional practice linked to the state of emergency,[9] what is striking at present is the lack/absence of work on what is happening internally and happens to us with the return to face-to-face sessions. As if the return to a "normal", known and established practice should not be a problem, should not hold any surprises.

In reality, the return of the real body to the session (that of the patient, but also that of we therapists) already entails, on a concrete level, the introduction of behaviours and acts subject to "external" norms that we are all obliged to comply with: the use of masks, the interpersonal distance to be maintained, the prohibition of any physical contact, the sanitisation of the rooms after each session, including the sanitisation of anything that may have been touched by the patient … sessions are no longer the place just "of two people talking in a room". The Government is present, as well the ghost of the COVID-19 virus.

As therapists, we have to be aware that for the patient we can now be heard as "possible carriers of the disease", no longer (or not only) as "the healers": the door of the practice has reopened, but it has allowed entry to fears, to persecutory and paranoid aspects, in which the therapist can be affected, lost, but can also be "the enemy", or convey the spread of the disease, like a careless and unobservant customs officer.

Z., a 73-year-old patient, in her third year of therapy, reveals these thoughts to me in a Skype session:

> I remembered a picture I saw years ago. It was a ship full of migrants, coming from Asia… mmm… that is, from Albania (she made a slip of the tongue) to Italy. It looked like an anthill swarming with beings, ready to assault our country.

In this sense, I believe that the decisions of some patients to continue their sessions online should be read, not only in rational terms as a facilitation, an optimisation and a saving of time, e.g., no longer having to commute to and from the therapist's office, but also as a tool that defends and protects the therapeutic bond, its positive, "good", healing value, keeps it safe; in the same way that seeing the patient, for example, on Skype has sometimes enabled us to discover his or her hitherto "silent" areas, so I believe that it may be the case for the return to usual practice.

I am well aware that I risk sounding like someone who has discovered something obvious: we all know, and very well, that every change in the setting entails a disruption! But it seems to me useful to recall in this regard what J. Bleger (1967) points out: when a patient begins psychotherapy, and encounters the setting proposed by his analyst, which refers to the therapist's own reference theories, precisely in this framework, in this ideally "normal" setting, his underlying unconscious fantasies remain silent. And it is not easy for the therapist to discover them since they do not become apparent until a break in the setting occurs. So perhaps it is in this sense that we should reflect on the experience as a whole, in patients and in ourselves.

With respect to how much the lockdown has also generated in our minds as therapists the "hut syndrome", forcing us to reconsider not only the way we act, but also the way we feel, and the effort involved in processing, which is indispensable to rebalance our internal structure and keep the function of the mind alive.

Conclusion

The incursion of the pandemic into our lives and into our daily work as psychoanalytic psychotherapists has not only undermined habits consolidated by many years of training and practice: the seesaw onto which the COVID-19 emergency has dragged us (first wave, lockdown, pseudo-normality, second wave, third wave, etc.) has challenged omnipotent beliefs and ideas, which in any case lurked within us, and which were partly linked to what scientific research has accustomed us to, namely that this problematic situation could be resolved, remedied and cured quickly, or that the problem could vanish on its own, just as it had arrived. This was not the case, and even the arrival of the vaccine was contemporaneous with the discovery of variants of the virus that were not very responsive to the vaccine itself. The time-frame to resolution thus became disproportionately long, and it was not always possible to reopen our offices after a fairly short interval.

This dilated and indefinite time has in fact multiplied the questions on which we must forcibly stop and reflect, on how we have kept and kept alive the thread of the therapeutic relationship with patients who have refused online work, and whom we have therefore not seen for so long; whether online sessions always retained their value, even over the long term, sometimes a year or more; with the patients we received in person, what the presence of the masks, not seeing each other's faces, entailed, especially in face-to-face psychotherapies, especially those initiated during the pandemic. And as psychotherapists, how did we deal with the illness and death of our patients?

There are indeed many questions that require our attention and rethinking, in these uncertain, anxiety-laden times, often metaphorically represented as times of war.

So, just as I wanted to start with Ferro's words, I would like to conclude by borrowing those of an anonymous analyst, referred to by S. Anastasia and R. Goisis (2020), which I found wonderful: "Bion comes to mind, his War Memories. I am helping my patients to write their War Memories. I am helping myself to write mine."

Notes

1 Antonino Ferro, interview with the newspaper *La Stampa*, 3 March 2013.
2 For example, the Youngle Project conceived and promoted by the Municipality of Florence and the Region of Tuscany as early as 2012 with social media chats and counselling, subsequently adopted in many other regions of Italy.
3 These notes certainly do not intend to, nor can they replace or exhaust the great debate that has raged on the subject of online psychoanalysis and psychoanalytic psychotherapy, but contribute, in their limited nature, to stimulating thoughts and reflections on the subject.
4 According to the writer W. Gibson, "cyberspace is the electronic space in which senses and brain are connected directly with the computer" (Marzi and Fiorentini, 2017).
5 I would like to thank S. Fano Cassese and A. Suman for discussing this point with me and helping me to better define my considerations.
6 The case of X. was followed by C. Pratesi.
7 Y.'s case was followed by L. Palchetti, whom we thank for allowing the use of the clinical material, taken from his postgraduate thesis.
8 Y.'s escape lasted four months, following rejection from school and a break of another four months due to the therapist's pregnancy.
9 Psychoanalysis gradually came into contact with the full drama of the situation. Gradually allowing itself to be infected by what was happening and organising its 'immune defences' so as not to make its patients ill … at the beginning of the pandemic, Donatella Lisciotto told everyone with sincerity that 'as the days went by, I stopped pretending not to listen to my anguish and I came to terms with a silent restlessness'. Various defence mechanisms have also been put in place internally: splitting, intellectualisation, repression, displacement, repression, denial, trivialisation. (Anastasia and Goisis, 2020)

References

Anastasia, S. and Goisis, R. (2020). Allarme. C'è un virus nella stanza! Un tentativo di ricostruzione delle primissime riflessioni psicoanalitiche sulle fasi precoce della pandemia. Available at: https://www.spiweb.it/cultura/allarme-ce-un-virus-nella-stanza-s-a nastasia-p-r-goisis/
Bleger, J. (1967). *Simbiosis y ambigüedad: estudio psicoanalitico*. Buenos Aires: Editorial Paidòs.
Bolognini, S. (2020). Riflessioni sulla pandemia. Available at: https://www.spiweb.it/wp content/uploads/2020/03/bolognini.pdf
Eiguer, A. (2004). *L'inconscient de la maison*. Paris: Dunod.
Fano Cassese, S. (2001). *Introduction to the Work of Donald Meltzer*. London: Karnac.

Ferro, A. (2013). Persone, personaggi, ologrammi. In A. Marzi (ed.), *Psicoanalisi, identità e Internet. Esplorazioni nel cyberspace.* Milan: FrancoAngeli.

Freud, S. (1905 [2001]). Three. In J. Strachey (ed.), *The Standard Edition of the Complete Psychological Works of Sigmund Freud.* London: Hogarth Press.

Lisciotto, D. (2020). Solo Voce. Available at: https://www.spiweb.it/wpcontent/uploads/2020/03/lisciotto.pdf

Marzi, A. and Fiorentini, G. (2017). Light and Shadow in Online Psychoanalysis. Available at: https://www.spiweb.it/wpcontent/uploads/2020/03/marzi-fiorentini.pdf

Micotti, S. (2020). Apprendere dall'esperienza Covid-19: prime riflessioni sul lavoro psicoanalitico online con le famiglie. Available at: http://www.saramicotti.com/apprendere-da llesperienza-covid-19-prime-riflessionisul-lavoro-psicoanalitico-online-con-le-famiglie/

Migone, P. (2003). La psicoterapia con Internet. *Psicoterapia e Scienze Umane,* XXXVII(4): 5773.

Nicolò, A.M. (2020). Introduzione della Presidente della SPI. Available at: https://www.spiweb.it/areadibattiti/analisi-e-psicoterapie-internet-o-per-telefono-al-tempo -del-coronavirus/

Nissim Momigliano, L. (1984). Due persone che parlano in una stanza. Una ricerca sul dialogo analitico. *Rivista di Psicoanalisi,* 30: 1–17.

Richard, F. (2020). Psicoanalisi a distanza: Skype o telefono? Available at: https://www.spiweb.it/wpcontent/uploads/2020/03/richard.pdf

Robutti, A. (2001). Introduzione. In L. Nissim Momigliano (ed.), *L'ascolto rispettoso. Scritti psicoanalitici.* Milan: Raffaello Cortina.

Saul, L.J. (1951). A Note on the Telephone as a Technical Aid. *Psychoanalytic Quarterly,* 20: 287–290.

Suman, A. (2022). *Psicoterapia psicoanalitica, percorsi geografici nella relazione terapeutica.* Paper presented at AFPP, Associazione Fiorentina di Psicoterapia Psicoanalitica, Florence, March 2022 (unpublished text).

Chapter 10

... and the door closes

Rethinking the session

Antonio Suman

Filling in absences

The psychotherapeutic session is the source of notations, information, emotional events that must be carefully examined and analysed; it is the subject of reflections, fantasies, of the patient as well as the therapist. But what happens to the therapist when the patient has left the therapy room? As far as the patient's thoughts about the session are concerned, he may communicate them to us spontaneously in the next meeting, or he may be invited to recount his experience of the previous session. When I ask, for example, "Do you ever think about our sessions during the week?", I am sometimes surprised by the communication of patients who report having reflected on a sentence of mine to which I had not given much importance. In general, I leave the incipit of the session to the patient, allowing him to communicate the point of emergence of his thoughts at that moment. However, I am also convinced that some "stitching-up" is necessary, giving a sense of continuity between sessions so that they become integrated. Unlike in psychoanalysis, in psychotherapy sessions take place with a variable frequency of once, twice a week and sometimes even every 15 days; in this sense, establishing a thread between one session and the next helps to keep the focus on the significant themes at work in the therapeutic relationship. The other important consequence is that the patient realises that when we refer to the previous session, we have not forgotten him on the days when he did not see us. This comment has a positive effect: it shows that we are really interested in the patient, and that we have thought about him.

Storytelling

I usually do not write during the session and, once it is concluded, the few minutes that follow are devoted to notes: sometimes only a few lines, other times, if important topics have been touched upon, I write a longer report, briefly noting the main topics discussed. I devote special space to the patient's dreams, when I have not transcribed them during the session itself. Dreams are sometimes long and confusing or are composed of successive sequences

DOI: 10.4324/9781032673721-11

that are more or less congruent and therefore not always easy to keep in mind in order to use them as the object of analysis. The report serves, in my opinion, to fix in my memory the themes dealt with in the previous session(s), but it also has the function of re-processing what has happened; that is, a re-reading of the events takes place, still under the emotional effect of the session, which I transcribe in a narrative manner. I find this a significant moment, but one that does not seem to have been given much consideration. The importance of writing lends itself to a reliving of the session with its cognitive, emotional, relational contents; it represents, beyond the recorded data, a sort of revisiting, almost on a dream level, of a narration that is not only a chronicle of what happened but opens up new perspectives or highlights some element of the material that perhaps I had not sufficiently considered.

Second-level rêverie or semi-dream position

Single-week sessions (or with longer intervals) lend themselves to being occupied by the patient's account of the events that have occurred during the past week; this is not bad in an absolute sense, but it reduces the possibility of reflecting on behaviour, thoughts and emotions that are not sufficiently processed, with the risk of a trivialisation of the relationship. The reality of the patient's experience does not become, to quote Bion (1962), "learning from experience".

By writing, we are not reproducing the reality of the session, but we are reconstructing our own representation of it, which also includes the notation of our feeling: we may have felt bored, rejected, powerless, excited, frustrated, satisfied, etc. Having nothing to write about means that therapy stagnates.

We may also realise how difficult it was to reach out to a patient who fears intimacy, or that we did not have sufficient restraint against the disruptive emotionality of a borderline subject, or that we unconsciously counter-identified with the patient when he used projective identification on a massive scale, etc. The critical review of the course of the session that has just ended may reveal aspects of the relationship that we had not noticed before.

A particular condition is that of the patient who comes regularly to the sessions and uses them to "discharge" all the anxieties, misadventures and frustrations that have happened to him during the week. Once the report is finished, the time of the session is exhausted and in the next one the picture repeats itself identically; the therapist's interventions are listened to, but nothing changes in the course of the therapy, nor in the daily life of the subject. It can be assumed that at the end of the session its contents are each time evacuated and thus erased, the session forgotten with the consequent sense of frustration on the part of the therapist. This stereotypical pattern is reminiscent of D. Meltzer's (1967) concept of the "toilet breast", which he describes as an early phase of psychoanalysis. It is probable that underlying this behaviour is a fear of establishing any kind of dependent relationship with the therapist.

One can rethink the session even without writing: after all, psychotherapy, too, is no less than psychoanalysis, "a process based on thinking and rethinking, dreaming and redreaming, discovering and rediscovering" (Ogden, 2009). The "therapist's dreaming" is a concept proposed by Ogden, who formulates it on the basis of psychoanalysis experiences with multi-week sessions. However, it is possible at many moments of psychotherapy to assume the same attitude. And if we find this activity difficult during a face-to-face session, it can be recovered later, when the patient has physically left the room but has left a silence and an empty space that we can fill – if we give ourselves the time – with our representations and answer the questions: and now what do I feel?, what do I think about this encounter?, what remains for me? I usually re-enact the entrance to the consulting room: did he look at me as usual or did he avoid me with his gaze? When the session ended, was his attitude different? Did he leave saying "thank you" to please me or because he actually felt helped? And was my reading of the dream told in the session a real help in clarifying certain anxieties of the patient and did it serve to better see the type of relationship at work? Do I realise, after the end of the session, that I missed a point in the conversation which I had not considered, and wonder why I did not see it? Does it represent a "blind spot" of mine and of what kind? Instead, am I satisfied with having made a good reconstruction of scattered elements of our conversation and thus succeeded in giving the communication a new, more integrated and more convincing meaning? When I have caught positive or negative transference references that the patient has accepted, has a new potential space opened up in which to continue working, has the relationship been consolidated? Basically, these are effects that are part of countertransference, of which one becomes aware only immediately after the session.

I would like to quote a passage by Franco Mori about the case of a psychotic patient who was locked in her silence for a very long time. The work has been republished in memory of his recent death in the journal *Contrappunto*:

> During the long period in which I used my hands to open Francesca's, it often happened to me after she had left to put them in front of my face and my sensitive nose. I would then sometimes inhale a subtle, pleasant smell, like healthy, fresh, clean skin, and I would tell myself that I was getting something from her after all. Something pleasant, that remained in me.
>
> (1993)

Ogden develops the concept of dreaming for the patient by stating that this kind of dreaming is to be imagined as "a second-level rêverie" as it is more organised and structured than the maternal rêverie. Furthermore, summarising Bion's thought, he writes: "The work of dreaming, for Bion, is the psychological work by which we create personal, symbolic meaning, thereby becoming ourselves" (2009).

He goes so far as to say that the purpose of the psychoanalytic (but, I would add, also psychoanalytic psychotherapeutic) process is to help the patient develop his capacity to think and feel his own experience. Once the process is initiated, the patient is in a position to begin to confront and come to an agreement with his or her emotional problems.

In this sense, it seems to me that there is a strong analogy between the function of the child's play that develops his capacity for symbolic representation and the waking dream activity of the adult that can be seen as playing with reality, that is, treating reality as a representation that can be processed in multiple aspects. Indeed, the child's play is not only the learning of useful skills but also has the function of processing the anxiety and emotional tensions of the moment. Thus, the development of oneiric capacity while awake activates representations that allow us to free ourselves from the bonds associated with discomfort and suffering and it is for this reason that I believe that the psychoanalytic therapist's dream can implement the patient's psychic life. The recovery of creativity increases the sense of personal worth.

In psychodynamic psychotherapy, this ability to play is central in order not to remain "flattened" in the recording of the facts reported by the patient.

Questions awaiting answers

I think an important part of the post-session time is about the questions I ask myself and to which I do not know, or perhaps do not yet know, how to give some answers. Any report is by nature unfinished, but putting it together can help us tolerate the sense of bewilderment in the face of not knowing.

References

Bion, W.R. (1962). *Learning from Experience*. London: W. Heinemann Medical Books.
Meltzer, D. (1967). *The Psychoanalytic Process*. London: W. Heinemann,
Mori, F. (1993). Quando difetta il linguaggio verbale nella coppia paziente terapeuta. *Contrappunto*, 59: 12–32.
Ogden, T.H. (2009). *Rediscovering Psychoanalysis: Thinking and Dreaming, Learning and Forgetting*. London: Routledge.

Index

Note to index: page numbers in *italics* refer to information in figures; page numbers in **bold** refer to information in tables.